The Australian Women's Weekly — Home Library

D0520003

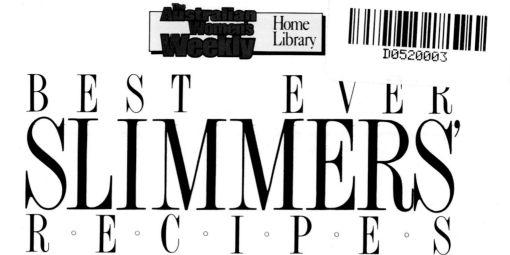

BEST EVER SLIMMERS' R·E·C·I·P·E·S

Now we've designed a cookbook that won't make you feel as if you're on a diet. The meals have been carefully planned so that you can steadily lose weight without feeling deprived and all you'll gain is energy and a sense of well-being.

There are about 200 recipes in the book, each made to serve 4, and half of these are main courses with the majority being below 1255 kilojoules (300 calories). Also included are soups, entrees, side dishes and enticing desserts so that you can easily plan meals for the family or for a dinner party.

As well as recipes for those keen to lose weight, we have considered non-meat eaters, cholesterol watchers and those on salt-reduced diets. Top nutritionist Rosemary Stanton has worked out a kilojoule and calorie count for each recipe as well as compiling a kilojoule/calorie counter in the centre of the book which can be removed for ready reference.

If you're not losing weight on your present diet, then this is the book for you.

Pamela Clark

FOOD EDITOR

Back Cover: Rare Roast Beef and Asparagus Salad page 79
Front Cover: Chocolate Baskets page 122
China: Limoges from Studio-Haus

Produced by The Australian Women's Weekly Special Projects Division.
Typeset by Photoset Computer Service Pty Ltd, Sydney, Australia
Printed by Dai Nippon Co Ltd, Tokyo, Japan
Published by Australian Consolidated Press, 54 Park Street, Sydney
Distributed by Network Distribution Company, 54 Park Street, Sydney

Best Ever Slimmers Recipes.
Includes index.
ISBN 0 949892 83 1.

1. Reducing diets — Recipes. I Title:
Australian Women's Weekly.

641.5'635

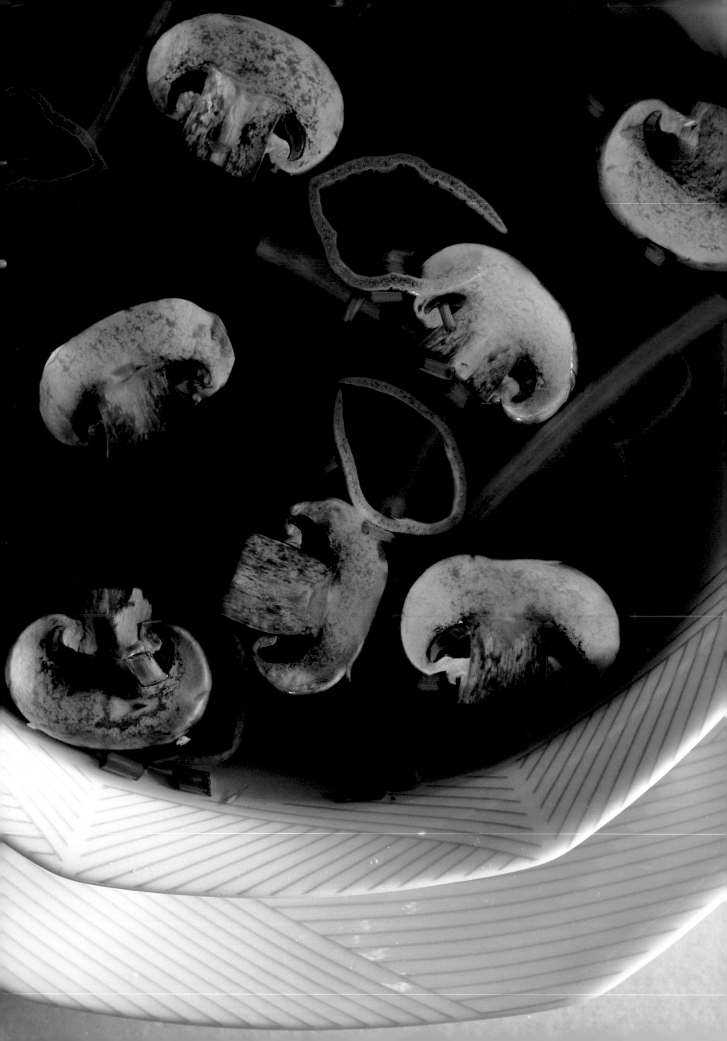

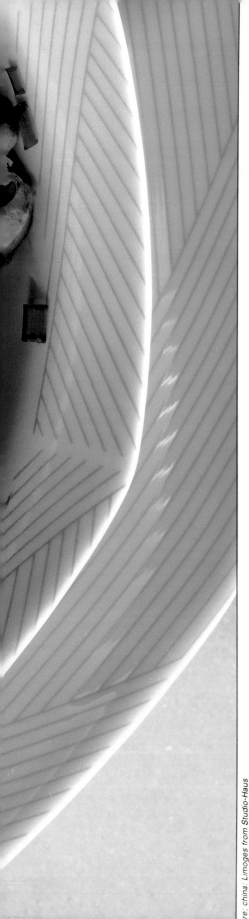

SOUPS

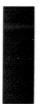

Many of our delicious soups can be made ahead of serving time and can be frozen until they are needed. Many can be cooked in the microwave oven, so they are quick to make, too. We have used stock cubes to add flavour but, if you prefer, you can make your own stock (see Glossary, page 124).

VEGETABLE CONSOMME

Stock can be prepared up to 2 days ahead, or frozen for up to 2 months. Recipe is not suitable to microwave.

2 large carrots (400g)
1 medium stick celery (80g)
8 cups water
1 tablespoon whole black
**   peppercorns**
2 cloves garlic, halved
2 bay leaves
1 large leek (250g), sliced
125g mushrooms, sliced
2 teaspoons light soya sauce
1 teaspoon dry sherry
1 small chicken stock cube,
**   crumbled**
1 tablespoon chopped fresh chives

Cut carrots and celery into thin strips; reserve any scraps. Combine water, peppercorns, garlic, bay leaves and carrot and celery scraps in a large saucepan. Bring to the boil, reduce heat, simmer, uncovered, 15 minutes. Strain, reserve stock; discard peppercorn mixture.

Return stock to saucepan, bring to the boil, add leek, reduce heat, simmer 5 minutes, add strips of carrot and celery, simmer 3 minutes. Add mushrooms, soya sauce, sherry and stock cube, simmer 1 minute. Stir in chives just before serving.

Serves 4.

Approximately 155 kilojoules (37 calories) per serve.

TOMATO HERB SOUP

This soup will thicken on standing; add a little water, if necessary. Soup can be frozen for up to 2 months. This recipe is not suitable to microwave.

1 bacon rasher (40g), chopped
1 medium onion (120g), chopped
1 clove garlic, crushed
2 cups water
1 small stick celery (60g), chopped
2 medium carrots (240g), finely
**   chopped**
425g can tomatoes
1 small chicken stock cube,
**   crumbled**
30g spaghetti
2 small zucchini (200g), chopped
1 tablespoon tomato paste
1 tablespoon chopped fresh basil
1 tablespoon chopped fresh parsley

Combine bacon, onion and garlic in a large saucepan, stir constantly over heat until onion is soft (or microwave on HIGH for about 5 minutes). Add water, celery, carrots, undrained crushed tomatoes and stock cube. Cover, bring to the boil, reduce heat, simmer 5 minutes (or microwave on HIGH for about 5 minutes). Add spaghetti and zucchini; simmer, uncovered, for about 10 minutes or until spaghetti is tender (or microwave on HIGH for about 10 minutes). Then stir in tomato paste, basil and parsley. Reheat before serving.

Serves 4.

Approximately 670 kilojoules (160 calories) per serve.

Table: Freedom Furniture; china: Limoges from Studio-Haus

Vegetable Consommé

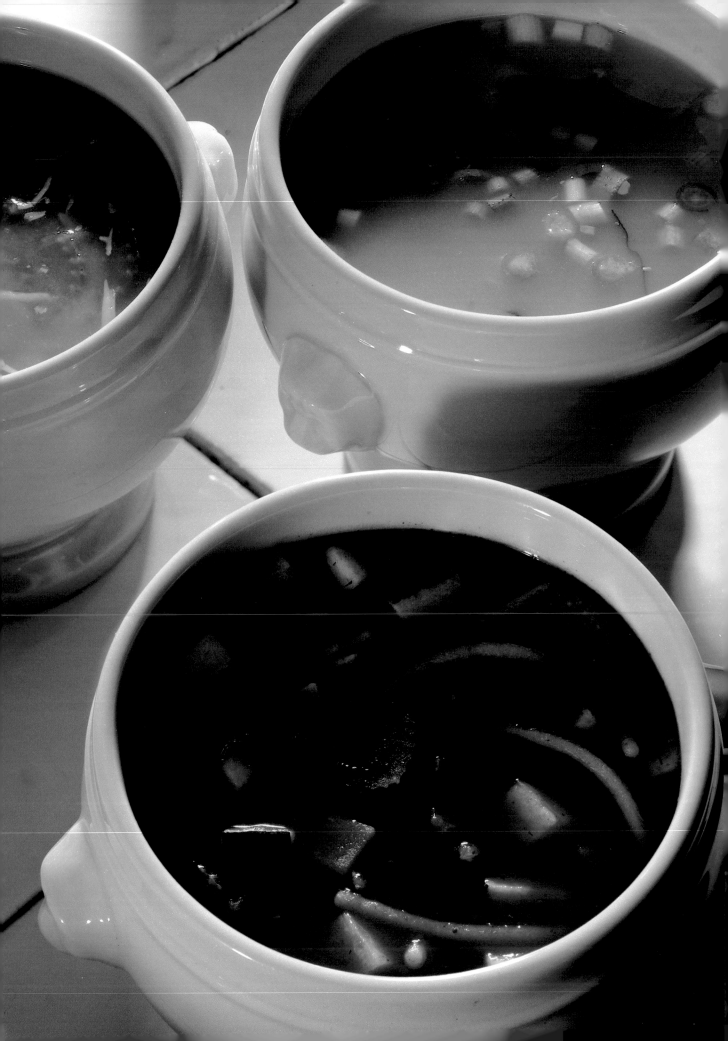

CREAMY CELERY SOUP

This recipe is not suitable to freeze or microwave.

8 small sticks celery (480g), thinly sliced
1 large onion (140g), finely chopped
3 cups water
1 tablespoon plain flour
1 small chicken stock cube, crumbled
2 tablespoons sour light cream
2 teaspoons grated parmesan cheese
1 tablespoon chopped fresh parsley
1 teaspoon lemon juice

Combine celery, onion and quarter cup of the water in a large saucepan, stir constantly over heat until onion is soft. Blend flour with another quarter cup of the water until smooth, stir into onion mixture, then stir in remaining water and stock cube. Stir constantly over heat until mixture boils and thickens. Reduce heat, simmer, covered, further 5 minutes. Stir in sour cream, cheese, parsley and lemon juice.

Serves 4.

 Approximately 215 kilojoules (50 calories) per serve.

CURRIED PUMPKIN SOUP

Soup can be made up to a day ahead; store, covered, in refrigerator. Soup can be frozen for up to 2 months. This recipe is not suitable to microwave.

1kg pumpkin, peeled
15g butter
1 medium onion (120g), chopped
2 teaspoons curry powder
¼ teaspoon ground cumin
1 litre (4 cups) water
1 small chicken stock cube, crumbled
1 tablespoon chopped fresh parsley

Chop pumpkin into small pieces. Heat butter in large saucepan, add onion, curry powder and cumin, stir constantly over heat until onion is soft. Add pumpkin, water and stock cube to saucepan, bring to the boil, reduce heat, simmer, covered, until pumpkin is tender. Blend or process pumpkin mixture until smooth. Stir in parsley.

Serves 4.

Approximately 325 kilojoules (77 calories) per serve.

CREAMED CORN SOUP

This recipe is not suitable to freeze.

310g can creamed corn
4 green shallots, chopped
2 cups water
1 small chicken stock cube, crumbled
½ teaspoon grated fresh ginger
1 egg, lightly beaten

Combine corn, shallots, water, stock cube and ginger in saucepan, bring to the boil, reduce heat, simmer, uncovered, for 2 minutes (or microwave on HIGH for about 5 minutes). Remove from heat, gradually whisk in egg; serve immediately.

Serves 4.

Approximately 360 kilojoules (85 calories) per serve.

HERB AND POTATO SOUP

Soup can be made a day ahead; store, covered, in refrigerator. Soup may be frozen for up to 2 months.

2 cups water
2 small chicken stock cubes, crumbled
3 medium potatoes (300g), chopped
2 green shallots, chopped
1 tablespoon chopped fresh parsley
1 tablespoon chopped fresh chives
¼ cup evaporated skim milk
pinch ground nutmeg

Combine water and stock cubes in a saucepan, add potatoes and shallots, bring to the boil, reduce heat, cover, simmer until potatoes are tender (or microwave on HIGH for approximately 10 minutes).

Blend or process potato mixture until smooth, return to saucepan, stir in the remaining ingredients, heat without boiling.

Serves 4.

 Approximately 310 kilojoules (74 calories) per serve.

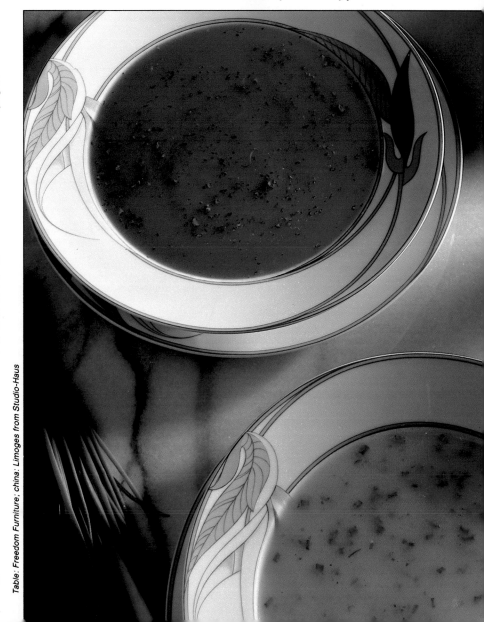

LEFT: Clockwise from left: Creamy Celery Soup; Creamed Corn Soup; Tomato Herb Soup. RIGHT: Top: Curried Pumpkin Soup; bottom: Herb and Potato Soup

Tiles: Pazotti; bowls: Pillivuyt from The Design Store

Table: Freedom Furniture; china: Limoges from Studio-Haus

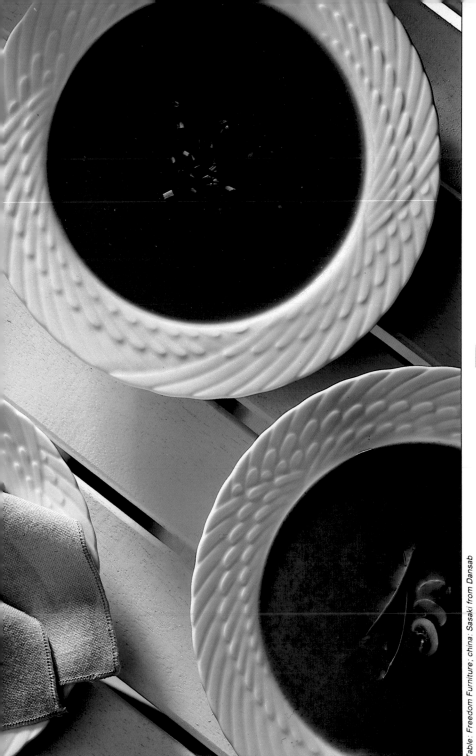

CREAMED MUSHROOM SOUP

Soup will keep, covered and refrigerated, for up to 2 days. It can be frozen for up to 2 months.

500g mushrooms
13g sachet low-joule vegetable soup mix
2 tablespoons dry sherry
2 cups water
1 tablespoon French mustard
1 tablespoon chopped fresh chives
2 tablespoons sour light cream

Combine mushrooms, soup mix, sherry, water, mustard in saucepan, cover, bring to the boil, reduce heat, simmer 10 minutes (or microwave on HIGH for about 10 minutes). Blend or process mushroom mixture until smooth, stir in chives and cream, reheat the soup before serving.
    Serves 4.

 Approximately 215 kilojoules (50 calories) per serve.

EASY CHILLED GAZPACHO

Soup can be made up to 2 days ahead; store, covered, in refrigerator. This recipe is not suitable to freeze.

3 medium cucumbers (840g), peeled, seeded, chopped
1 small red pepper (100g), chopped
1 small onion (80g), chopped
1 small stick celery (60g), chopped
1 small chilli, seeded, finely chopped
425g can tomatoes
1 clove garlic, crushed
⅓ cup No Oil French dressing
1 cup water
2 tablespoons chopped fresh parsley

Blend or process all ingredients until finely chopped, cover; refrigerate several hours or overnight before serving.
    Serves 4.

 Approximately 240 kilojoules (57 calories) per serve.

CHILLED CUCUMBER AND YOGHURT SOUP

Soup can be made up to 2 days ahead; store, covered, in refrigerator. Stir in yoghurt just before serving. This recipe is not suitable to freeze.

2 medium cucumbers (560g), peeled, seeded, chopped
1 medium pear (150g), chopped
1 gherkin (30g), chopped
200g carton low-fat plain yoghurt
1½ cups water
1 small chicken stock cube, crumbled
¼ cup fresh mint leaves

Blend or process all ingredients until smooth. Cover, refrigerate several hours before serving.
    Serves 4.

 Approximately 255 kilojoules (60 calories) per serve.

Table: Freedom Furniture; china: Sasaki from Dansab

FRESH TOMATO SOUP

Soup can be made a day ahead; store, covered, in refrigerator. If desired, 2 x 425g cans of tomatoes may be substituted for fresh tomatoes. This recipe is not suitable to freeze.

1 medium onion (120g), chopped
1 large carrot (200g), chopped
3 cups water
5 medium tomatoes (500g), peeled, chopped
1 small chicken stock cube, crumbled
2 tablespoons tomato paste
1 tablespoon chopped fresh chives

Combine onion and carrot in saucepan with quarter cup of the water. Stir constantly over heat until onion is soft (or microwave on HIGH for about 5 minutes). Add tomatoes (drained and crushed if using canned tomatoes), cover, simmer for 5 minutes. Add remaining water and stock cube, simmer 3 minutes (or microwave on HIGH for about 5 minutes). Blend or process tomato mixture until smooth, stir in tomato paste; sprinkle with chives.
    Serves 4.

 Approximately 255 kilojoules (60 calories) per serve.

ABOVE: Top: Fresh Tomato Soup; bottom: Creamed Mushroom Soup. RIGHT: Clockwise from left: Chilled Cucumber and Yoghurt Soup; Chilled Beetroot Soup; Easy Chilled Gazpacho.

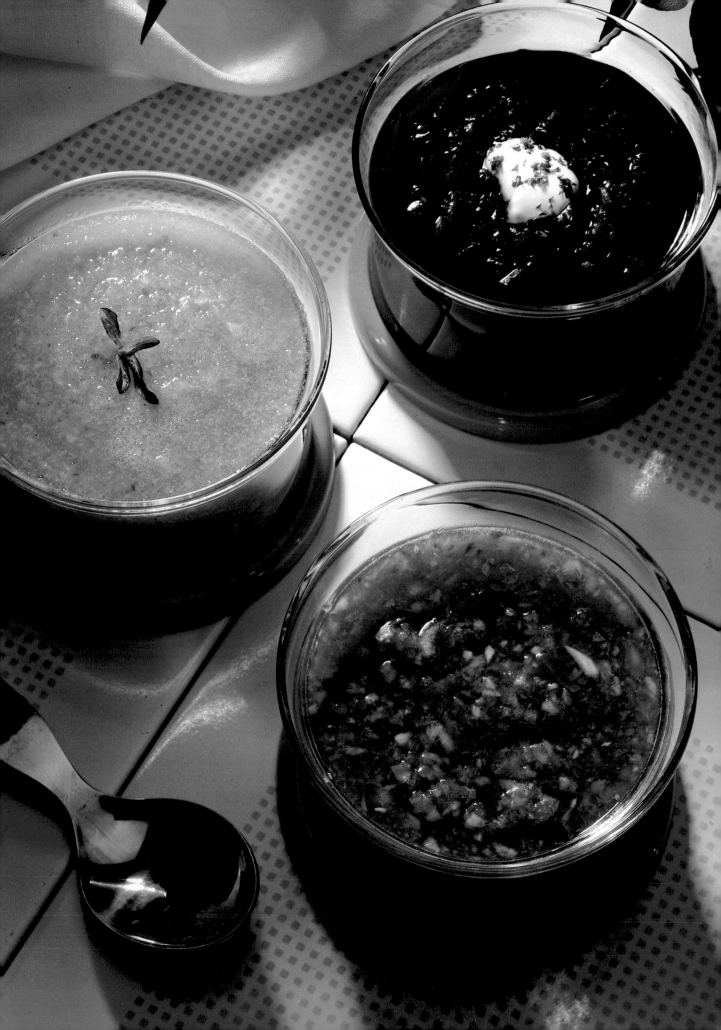

CHILLED BEETROOT SOUP

Soup can be made up to 2 days ahead; store, covered, in refrigerator. This recipe is not suitable to freeze.

3 large beetroot (500g)
2 medium cucumbers (560g), peeled, seeded, grated
1 small onion (80g), grated
1 small chicken stock cube, crumbled
3 cups water
2 tablespoons chopped fresh parsley
200g carton low-fat plain yoghurt

Place whole beetroot in saucepan, cover with cold water, cover saucepan, bring to the boil, reduce heat, simmer until beetroot are tender. Cooking time will depend on the size of the beetroot. Drain beetroot, cool, peel and grate into large bowl. Add cucumbers, onion, stock cube, water and parsley to beetroot. Cover, refrigerate several hours or overnight; top with yoghurt just before serving.

Serves 4.

 Approximately 345 kilojoules (82 calories) per serve.

BROCCOLI CAULIFLOWER SOUP

This recipe is not suitable to freeze.

500g broccoli
250g cauliflower
1 medium onion (120g), chopped
1 clove garlic, crushed
2 cups water
1 small chicken stock cube, crumbled
1 medium potato (100g), chopped
2 small sticks celery (120g), chopped
½ teaspoon dried marjoram leaves
1 cup skim milk
1 tablespoon chopped fresh parsley

Cut broccoli and cauliflower into flowerets. Combine onion and garlic in a large saucepan with 1 tablespoon of the water, stir constantly over heat until onion is soft (or microwave on HIGH for about 5 minutes). Add remaining water, stock cube, potato, celery, broccoli and cauliflower. Bring to the boil, reduce heat, simmer for 10 minutes or until potato is tender (or microwave on HIGH for about 10 minutes). Add marjoram. Blend or process broccoli mixture until smooth. Return to pan, add milk and parsley, reheat just before serving.

Serves 4.

 Approximately 375 kilojoules (90 calories) per serve.

ASPARAGUS CREAM SOUP

Soup can be made up to 2 days ahead; store, covered, in refrigerator. Or it can be frozen for up to 2 months.

1 teaspoon butter
1 small onion (80g), chopped
1 teaspoon plain flour
425g can asparagus cuts, drained
2 small chicken stock cubes, crumbled
2½ cups water
¼ cup evaporated skim milk
1 tablespoon sour light cream
1 teaspoon chopped fresh chives

Melt butter in saucepan, add onion; cook, stirring, until onion is soft (or microwave on HIGH for about 5 minutes). Stir in flour; cook 1 minute, stirring, then add asparagus, stock cubes and water. Bring to the boil, reduce heat, simmer, covered, for 5 minutes (or microwave on HIGH for about 5 minutes). Blend or process asparagus mixture until smooth, return to pan, add milk, heat without boiling. Stir in sour cream and sprinkle with chives just before serving.

Serves 4.

 Approximately 240 kilojoules (57 calories) per serve.

CURRIED CARROT SOUP

Soup can be made up to 2 days ahead; store, covered, in refrigerator. Or it can be frozen for up to 2 months.

2 medium carrots (240g), chopped
1 small onion (80g), chopped
1 small potato (75g), chopped
2 cups water
1 clove garlic, crushed
1 small chicken stock cube, crumbled
2 tablespoons orange juice
2 teaspoons curry powder
1 tablespoon tomato paste
1 cup skim milk
1 tablespoon chopped fresh parsley

Combine carrots, onion, potato, water, garlic and stock cube in large saucepan. Bring to the boil, reduce heat, simmer, covered, for 5 minutes or until vegetables are tender. Add orange juice, curry powder, tomato paste and skim milk. Blend or process carrot mixture until smooth. Return to pan, add parsley, reheat without boiling.

Serves 4.

Approximately 290 kilojoules (70 calories) per serve.

CHICKEN AND HAM SOUP

This recipe is not suitable to freeze.

1 chicken breast fillet (115g), sliced
2 medium zucchini (300g), sliced
30g baby mushrooms, sliced

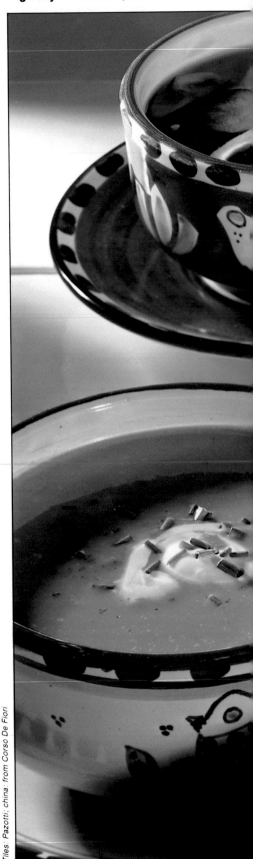

RIGHT: Clockwise from top left: Chicken and Ham Soup; Curried Carrot Soup; Broccoli Cauliflower Soup; Asparagus Cream Soup

Tiles: Pazotti; china: from Corso De Fiori

30g ham, sliced
2 green shallots, chopped
1 small chicken stock cube, crumbled
2 cups water
2 teaspoons light soya sauce
1 teaspoon cornflour

Combine chicken, zucchini, mushrooms, ham, shallots, stock cube and water in large saucepan. Bring to the boil, reduce heat, simmer, uncovered, for 5 minutes (or microwave on HIGH for about 5 minutes). Blend soya sauce with cornflour, add to pan, stir constantly over heat until soup boils and thickens slightly (or microwave soup on HIGH for about 3 minutes). Serve soup immediately.

Serves 4.

Approximately 200 kilojoules (48 calories) per serve.

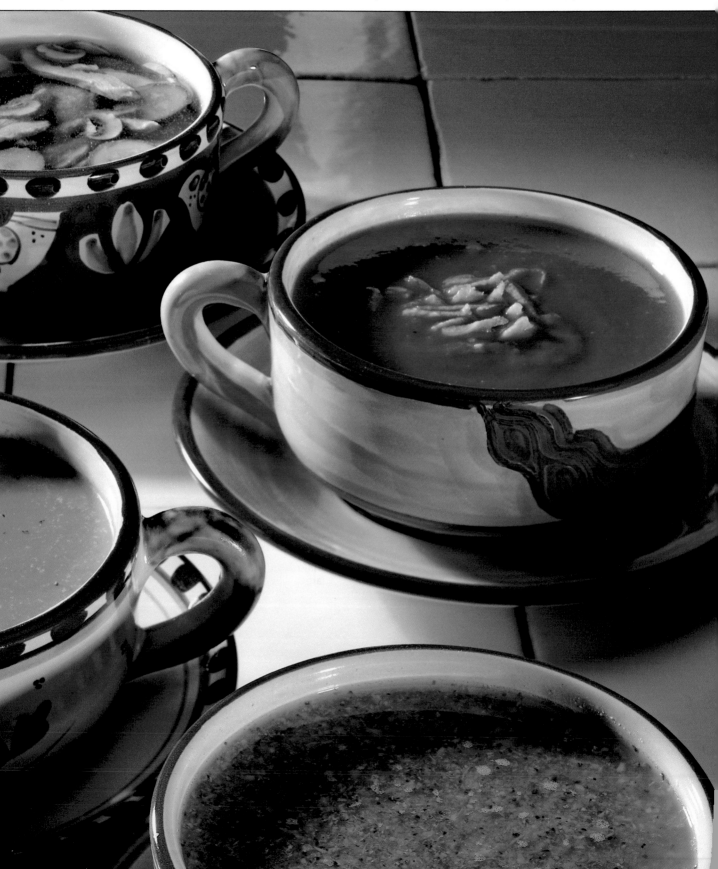

ENTREES

Our tempting entrees are special enough to serve at a dinner party where guests are counting the kilojoules. As many of the recipes do not contain any meat, they are more economical with kilojoules, making it possible for you to splurge a little with main course and dessert. The recipes also make ideal light lunches or snacks.

Dresser: Freedom Furniture; china: Mikasa

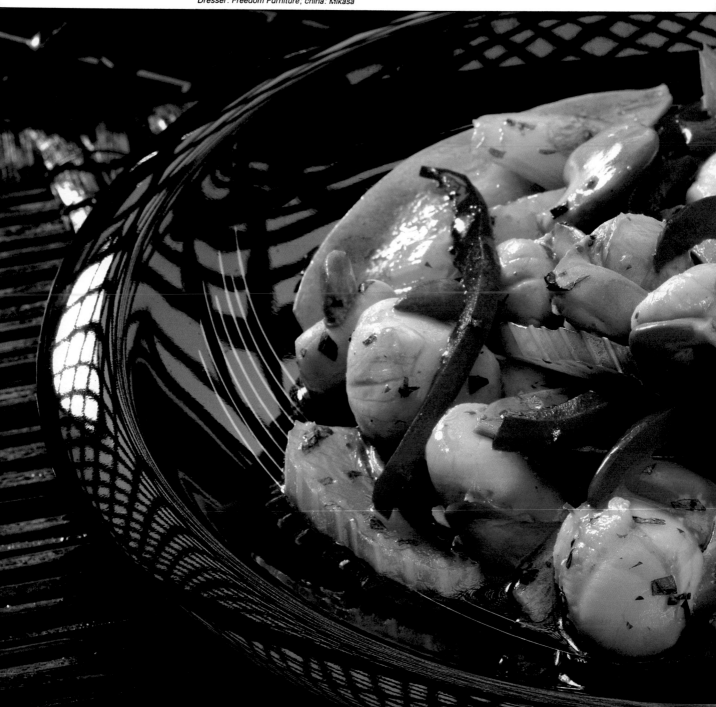

HONEYED SCALLOP AND CHILLI STIR-FRY

This recipe is not suitable to freeze or microwave.

3 teaspoons oil
1 medium onion (120g), quartered
2 medium red peppers (300g), thinly sliced
1 large stick celery (100g), sliced
100g snow peas
200g scallops
1 tablespoon honey
1 teaspoon chilli sauce
2 teaspoons chopped fresh mint

Heat oil in frying pan or wok, add vegetables to pan, stir-fry over high heat for about .1 minute. Add scallops, honey, chilli sauce and mint to pan, stir-fry for about 2 minutes or until scallops are tender.
    Serves 4.

Approximately 560 kilojoules (133 calories) per serve.

MARINATED SALMON AND AVOCADO SALAD

This recipe is not suitable to freeze.

½ medium avocado (100g)
100g smoked salmon
1 medium onion (120g), thinly sliced
125g cherry tomatoes, halved
4 mignonette lettuce leaves

MARINADE

1 tablespoon white vinegar
1 tablespoon lemon juice
3 teaspoons oil
1 clove garlic, crushed
2 teaspoons drained capers, chopped
2 teaspoons chopped fresh parsley
½ teaspoon sugar
¼ teaspoon dry mustard

Chop avocado, cut salmon into strips. Combine avocado, salmon, onion and tomatoes in bowl, add marinade. Cover, refrigerate 1 hour before serving; serve in lettuce leaves.
Marinade: Combine all ingredients in screw-top jar; shake well.
    Serves 4.

Approximately 585 kilojoules (140 calories) per serve.

Honeyed Scallop and Chilli Stir-Fry

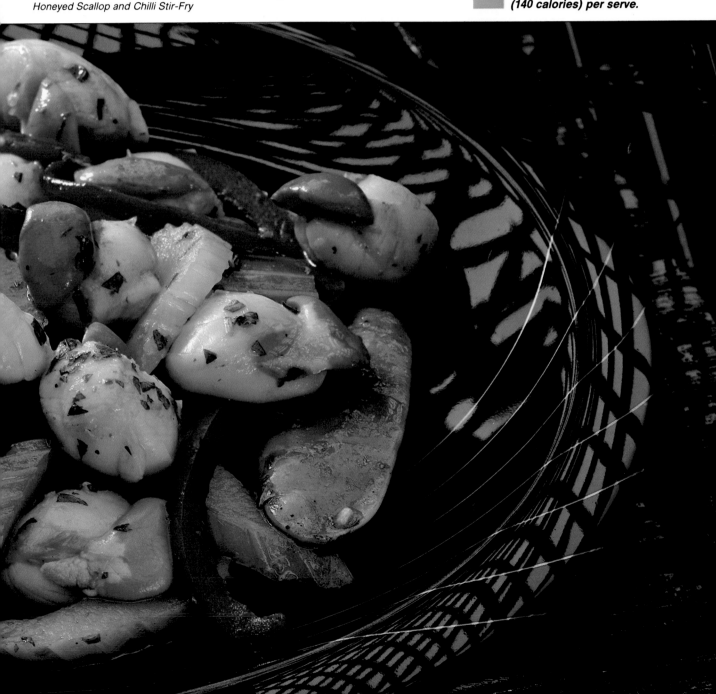

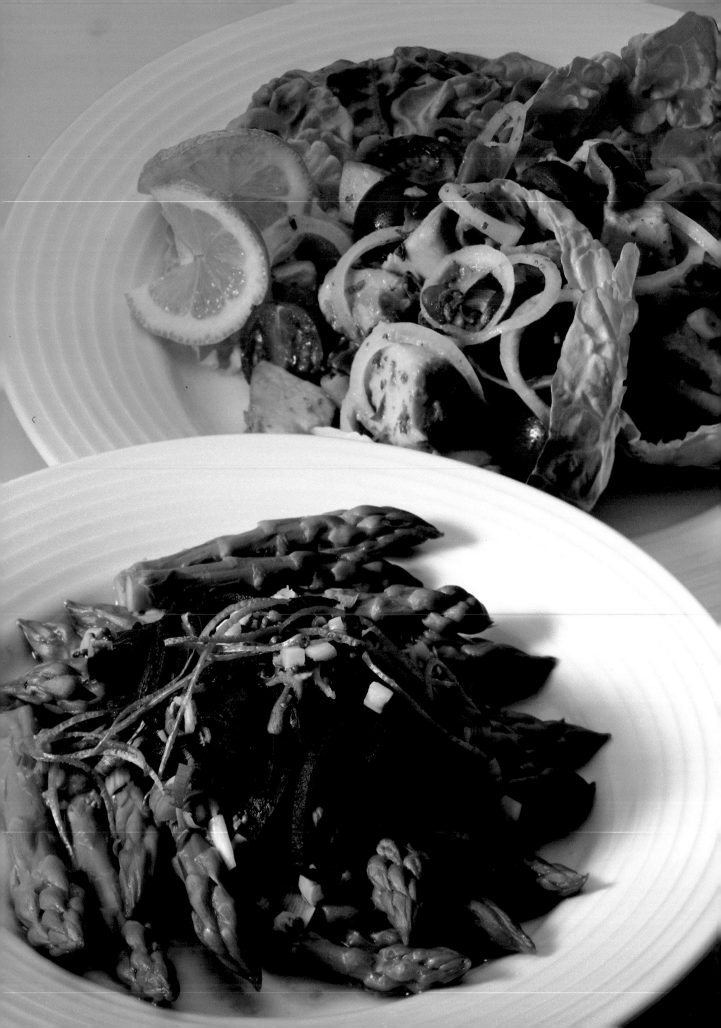

BEETROOT ASPARAGUS SALAD

This recipe is not suitable to freeze.

3 large fresh beetroot (500g)
24 fresh asparagus spears
DRESSING
2 tablespoons lemon juice
1 tablespoon orange juice
1 green shallot, chopped
½ teaspoon grated fresh ginger
½ teaspoon honey
1 teaspoon seeded mustard

Boil, steam or microwave whole, unpeeled beetroot until tender; drain, cool. Peel beetroot, cut into thin strips. Peel asparagus with vegetable peeler, boil, steam or microwave until just tender; drain, rinse under cold water, cut into 3 pieces. Place beetroot and asparagus on serving plate, top with dressing just before serving.
Dressing: Combine all ingredients in screw top jar; shake well.

Serves 4.

Approximately 270 kilojoules (65 calories) per serve.

CARROT MOUSSE WITH TOMATO SAUCE

This recipe is not suitable to freeze.

4 medium carrots (480g), chopped
2 teaspoons grated fresh ginger
¼ cup wholemeal plain flour
1 cup evaporated skim milk
3 eggs, lightly beaten
¼ teaspoon ground nutmeg
2 tablespoons chopped fresh chives
TOMATO SAUCE
425g can tomatoes
2 teaspoons cornflour
2 teaspoons sugar
1 tablespoon water

Boil, steam or microwave carrots until tender, drain. Blend or process carrots and ginger until smooth. Blend flour in a small saucepan with milk, stir constantly over heat until mixture boils and thickens (or microwave on HIGH about 3 minutes). Remove from heat; add to processor with eggs and nutmeg; process until smooth, stir in chives.

Pour mixture into 4 lightly greased 1 cup ovenproof dishes, place dishes into a baking dish. Pour in enough hot water to come halfway up sides of dishes, cover with foil. Bake in moderate oven for about 45 minutes or until set (or microwave, covered, on MEDIUM LOW for about 6 minutes). Turn onto serving plates, serve with tomato sauce.
Tomato Sauce: Blend or process undrained tomatoes until smooth, strain. Combine tomato in a saucepan with blended cornflour, sugar and water, stir constantly over heat until mixture boils and thickens (or microwave on HIGH for about 3 minutes).

Serves 4.

Approximately 400 kilojoules (95 calories) per serve.

GLAZED SPINACH MOUSSE

This recipe is not suitable to freeze.

30 English spinach leaves
1 medium carrot (120g), finely grated
1 large potato (185g)
1 medium onion (120g), finely chopped
¼ teaspoon ground nutmeg
2 eggs, lightly beaten
½ cup low-fat plain yoghurt
2 tablespoons grated parmesan cheese
SAUCE
½ x 13g sachet low-joule vegetable soup mix
½ cup water

LEFT: Top: Marinated Salmon and Avocado Salad; bottom: Beetroot Asparagus Salad. BELOW: Top: Carrot Mousse with Tomato Sauce; bottom: Glazed Spinach Mousse

Lightly grease 4 dishes (three-quarter cup capacity); line bases with greaseproof or baking paper.

Boil, steam or microwave spinach until tender, drain, squeeze out as much liquid as possible, chop spinach roughly. Combine spinach, carrot, potato and onion in bowl, stir in nutmeg, eggs, yoghurt and cheese; spoon into prepared dishes. Place dishes in a baking dish with enough hot water to come halfway up sides of dishes.

Cover dishes with foil, bake in moderate oven for about 1 hour or until set. Stand 10 minutes before turning onto serving plates; serve with sauce.
Sauce: Combine soup mix and water in a saucepan, stir constantly over heat until mixture boils and thickens.

Serves 4.

Approximately 695 kilojoules (166 calories) per serve.

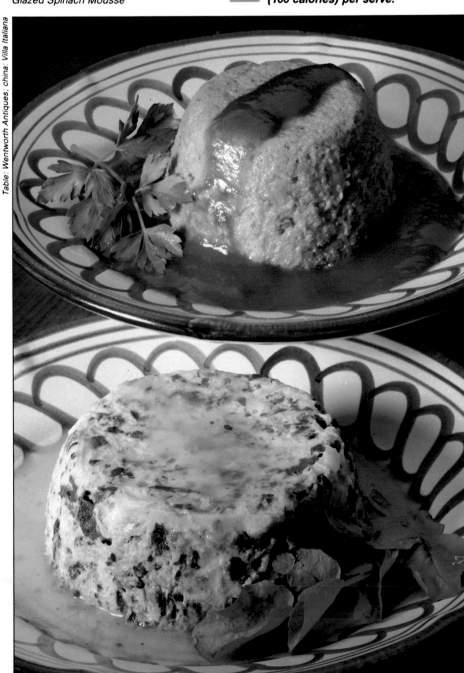

CITRUS CHICKEN KEBABS

Soak the skewers in water for about an hour to prevent burning during cooking. Recipe not suitable to freeze.

3 x 115g chicken breast fillets
2 tablespoons No Oil French dressing
2 teaspoons grated parmesan cheese
1 tablespoon orange juice
1 tablespoon lemon juice
1 tablespoon water
2 tablespoons chopped fresh basil
2 tablespoons chopped fresh parsley
3 green shallots, chopped

Cut chicken into 2cm pieces. Combine dressing, cheese, juices, water, basil, parsley, shallots and chicken in bowl, cover, refrigerate for 1 hour.

Thread chicken onto skewers. Grill on both sides, basting frequently with marinade (or microwave on HIGH for about 2 minutes).

Serves 4.

Approximately 690 kilojoules (165 calories) per serve.

SPICY SATAY STICKS

Sambal oelek is finely minced chillies, available in jars at supermarkets. For the best results refrigerate satays on their skewers before grilling. Satay sticks can be frozen, uncooked, for up to a month. This recipe is not suitable to microwave.

250g minced steak
1 teaspoon grated fresh ginger
2 small fresh red chillies, finely chopped
1 teaspoon turmeric
3 green shallots, chopped
1 clove garlic, crushed
2 teaspoons oil
1 teaspoon curry powder
SATAY SAUCE
3 green shallots, chopped
1 teaspoon sambal oelek
¼ cup crunchy peanut butter
1 tablespoon lemon juice
¼ cup water

Process all ingredients until finely minced. Divide mixture into 8 portions, mould each portion firmly around half of a bamboo skewer. Grill until golden brown and cooked through, turning once during cooking. Serve hot with satay sauce.

Satay Sauce: Combine shallots, sambal oelek, peanut butter, lemon juice and water in saucepan, stir until combined and heated through.

Serves 4.

Approximately 990 kilojoules (236 calories) per serve.

BELOW: Left: Citrus Chicken Kebabs; right: Spicy Satay Sticks. RIGHT: Spinach-Wrapped Chicken with Curry Sauce

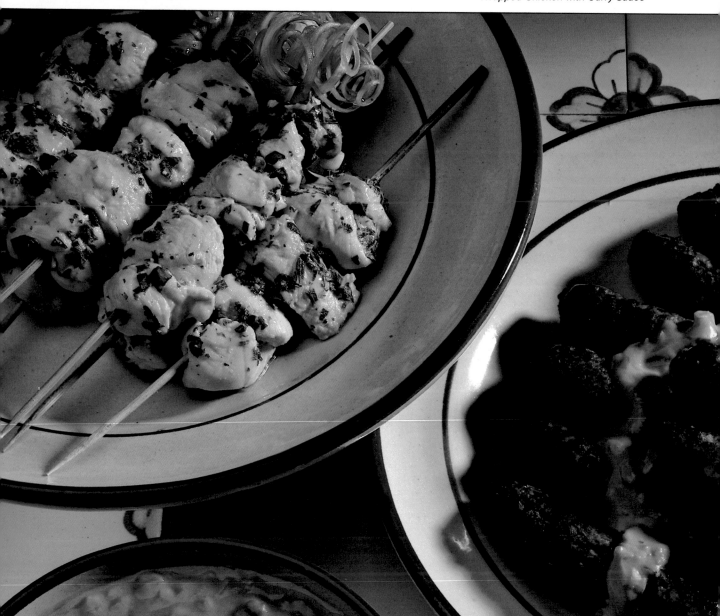

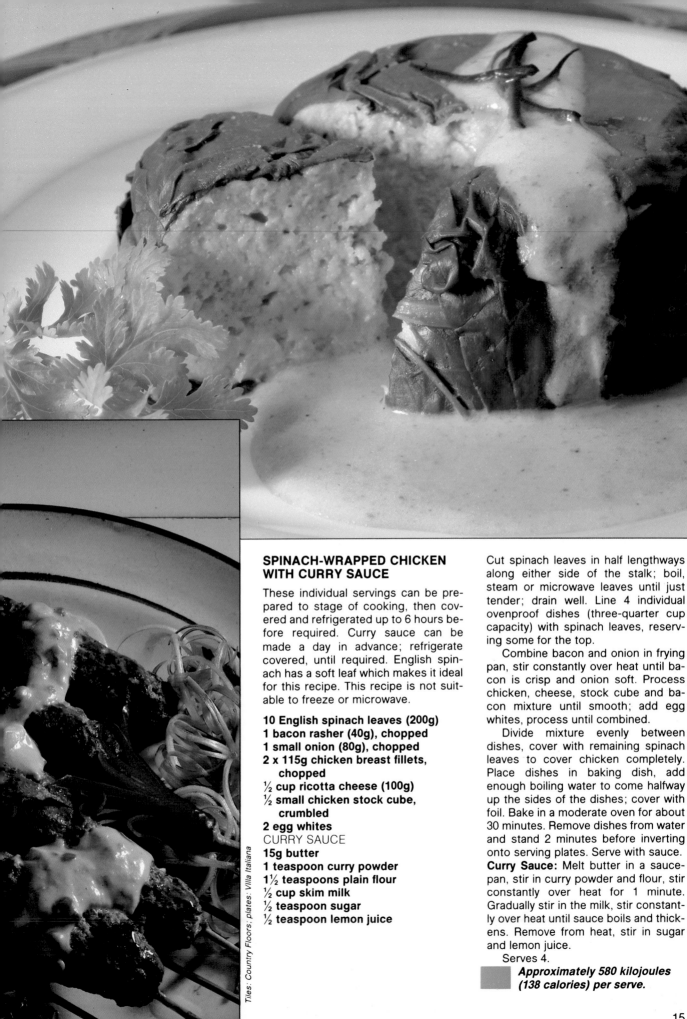

SPINACH-WRAPPED CHICKEN WITH CURRY SAUCE

These individual servings can be prepared to stage of cooking, then covered and refrigerated up to 6 hours before required. Curry sauce can be made a day in advance; refrigerate covered, until required. English spinach has a soft leaf which makes it ideal for this recipe. This recipe is not suitable to freeze or microwave.

10 English spinach leaves (200g)
1 bacon rasher (40g), chopped
1 small onion (80g), chopped
2 x 115g chicken breast fillets,
  chopped
½ cup ricotta cheese (100g)
½ small chicken stock cube,
  crumbled
2 egg whites
CURRY SAUCE
15g butter
1 teaspoon curry powder
1½ teaspoons plain flour
½ cup skim milk
½ teaspoon sugar
½ teaspoon lemon juice

Cut spinach leaves in half lengthways along either side of the stalk; boil, steam or microwave leaves until just tender; drain well. Line 4 individual ovenproof dishes (three-quarter cup capacity) with spinach leaves, reserving some for the top.

Combine bacon and onion in frying pan, stir constantly over heat until bacon is crisp and onion soft. Process chicken, cheese, stock cube and bacon mixture until smooth; add egg whites, process until combined.

Divide mixture evenly between dishes, cover with remaining spinach leaves to cover chicken completely. Place dishes in baking dish, add enough boiling water to come halfway up the sides of the dishes; cover with foil. Bake in a moderate oven for about 30 minutes. Remove dishes from water and stand 2 minutes before inverting onto serving plates. Serve with sauce.

Curry Sauce: Melt butter in a saucepan, stir in curry powder and flour, stir constantly over heat for 1 minute. Gradually stir in the milk, stir constantly over heat until sauce boils and thickens. Remove from heat, stir in sugar and lemon juice.

Serves 4.

Approximately 580 kilojoules (138 calories) per serve.

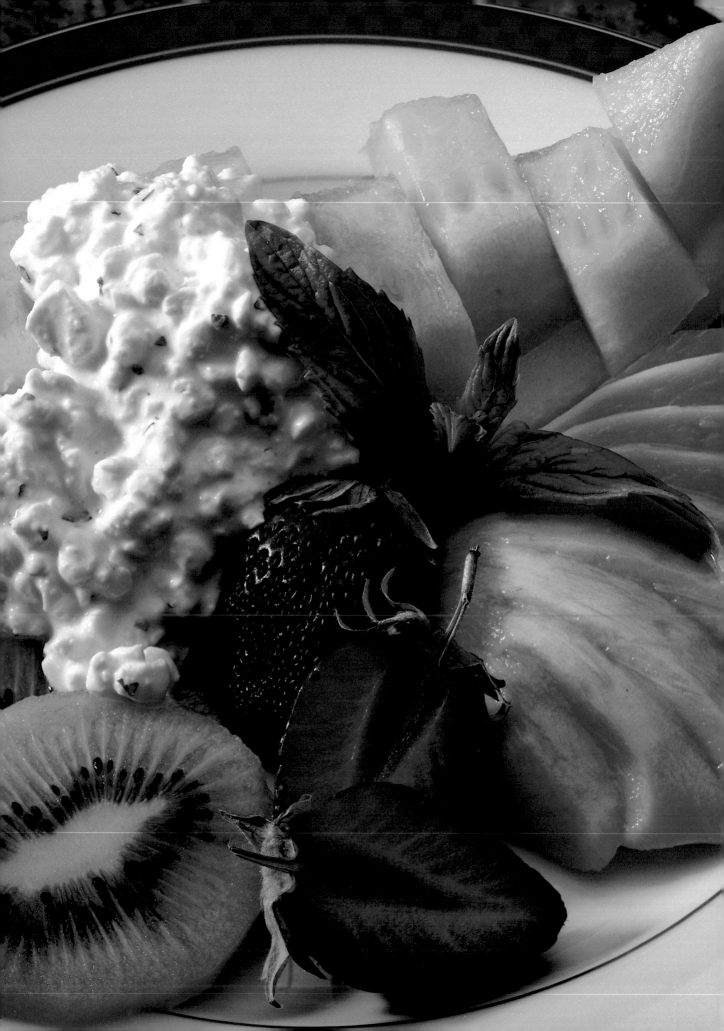

MINTED HONEY COTTAGE CHEESE WITH FRUIT

This recipe is not suitable to freeze.

250g carton low-fat cottage cheese
1 teaspoon honey
1 teaspoon finely chopped fresh mint
1 small honeydew melon (600g),
quartered
2 passionfruit
1 medium kiwi fruit (100g), sliced
1 small mango (200g), quartered
8 strawberries (75g)

Combine cottage cheese, honey and mint in bowl; mix well. Divide melon equally between plates and top with equal portions of cottage cheese mixture and passionfruit pulp. Divide fruit equally and arrange on plates.
    Serves 4.

Approximately 565 kilojoules (135 calories) per serve.

LEFT: Minted Honey Cottage Cheese with Fruit. BELOW: Top: Tasty Tuna Mousse; bottom: Salmon Mousse with Lemon and Chives

TASTY TUNA MOUSSE

This recipe is not suitable to freeze.

185g can tuna in brine, drained
2 tablespoons low oil mayonnaise
2 tablespoons lemon juice
1 small onion (80g), finely chopped
1 gherkin (30g), finely chopped
1 tablespoon chopped fresh parsley
1 tablespoon tomato paste
½ teaspoon dry mustard
¼ teaspoon sugar
3 teaspoons gelatine
2 tablespoons water

Blend or process tuna, mayonnaise, lemon juice, onion and gherkin until smooth. Add parsley, tomato paste, mustard and sugar, process until combined. Sprinkle gelatine over water, dissolve over hot water (or microwave on HIGH for about 20 seconds). Stir into tuna mixture.

    Rinse 4 individual half cup capacity dishes; do not dry dishes. Divide mixture evenly between dishes; cover, refrigerate several hours or overnight.

Approximately 360 kilojoules (85 calories) per serve.

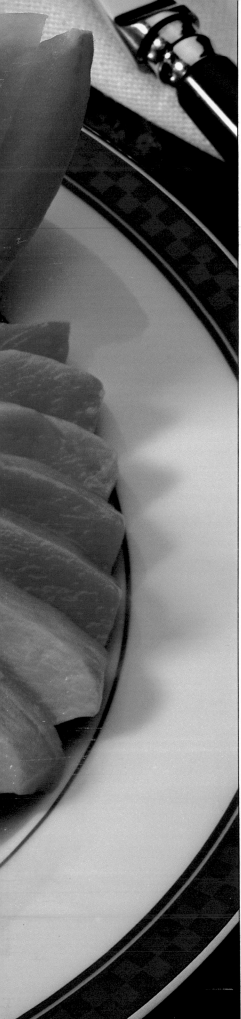

China: Noritake; fork and napkin: Studio-Haus
China: Noritake

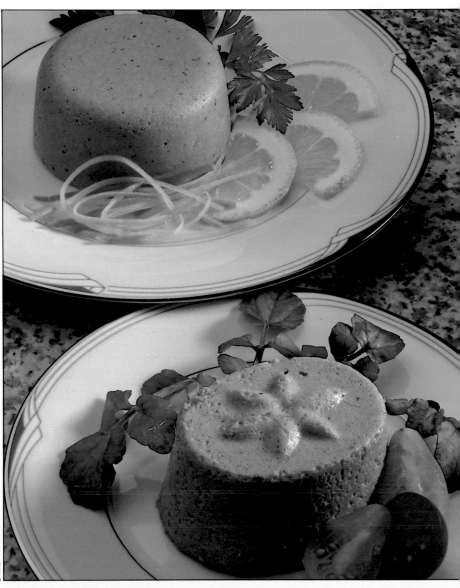

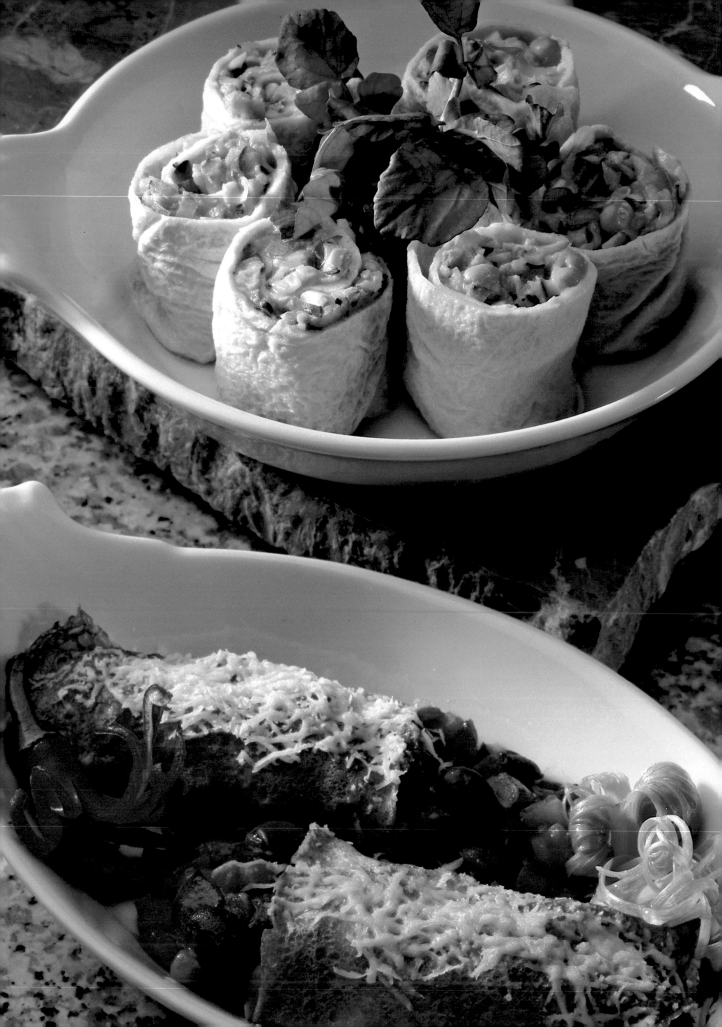

SALMON MOUSSE WITH LEMON AND CHIVES

This recipe is not suitable to freeze.

210g can red salmon, drained
1 medium stick celery (80g), chopped
2 teaspoons lemon juice
2 teaspoons low-fat, plain yoghurt
1 tablespoon chopped fresh chives
3 teaspoons gelatine
2 tablespoons water
¼ cup evaporated skim milk
1 egg white

Blend or process salmon, celery, lemon juice and yoghurt until smooth. Place mixture into bowl, stir in chives. Sprinkle gelatine over water, dissolve over hot water (or microwave on HIGH for about 20 seconds). Stir into salmon mixture. Stir milk into salmon mixture. Whisk egg white until firm peaks form; fold into salmon mixture.

Rinse 4 individual half cup capacity dishes; do not dry dishes. Divide mousse evenly between dishes; cover, refrigerate several hours or overnight.

Serves 4.

Approximately 555 kilojoules (132 calories) per serve.

ZUCCHINI AND AVOCADO OMELET ROLLS

Omelets and zucchini can be cooked up to 1 hour ahead. Fresh or canned corn kernels can be used. This recipe is not suitable to freeze.

OMELET
4 eggs
⅓ cup water
FILLING
2 medium zucchini (300g), grated
¼ large avocado (80g)
½ cup corn kernels
4 green shallots, chopped

Whisk eggs and water together in a small bowl. Heat a small frying pan, grease lightly. Pour 1½ tablespoons of egg mixture into pan; use an egg slide to push edges of omelet towards the centre so omelet becomes a round shape, about 12cm in diameter. When omelet is just set but still a little creamy on top, carefully remove from pan, using an egg slide. Repeat with remaining mixture to make 8 omelets.

Spread filling onto omelets, roll up. Place rolls onto an oven tray. Bake, uncovered, in moderate oven for about 5 minutes or until slightly warm (or microwave on MEDIUM for about 1½ minutes). Cut each omelet into 3 pieces before serving.

Filling: Place zucchini in pan, cover, cook until just tender (or microwave on HIGH for about 2 minutes). Drain zucchini well, press out as much liquid as possible. Mash avocado in bowl, stir in zucchini, corn and shallots.

Serves 4.

Approximately 625 kilojoules (150 calories) per serve.

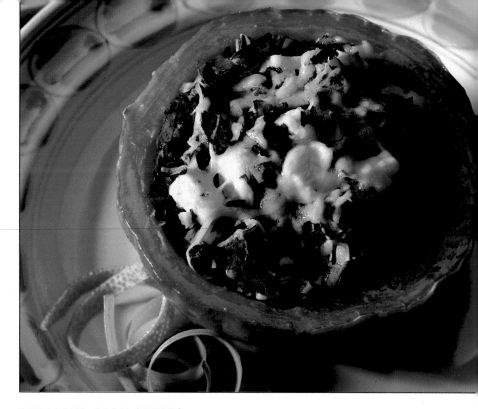

CHILLI AND CORN CREPES

Filling can be made one day before required. Recipe unsuitable to freeze.

CREPES
¼ cup plain flour
1 egg, lightly beaten
½ cup skim milk
½ teaspoon oil
FILLING
310g can red kidney beans, rinsed, drained
130g can corn kernels, drained
1 small red pepper (100g), finely chopped
1 small green pepper (100g), finely chopped
1 small onion (80g), finely chopped
1 small fresh red chilli, finely chopped
425g can tomatoes
¼ cup dry red wine
1 tablespoon cornflour
1 tablespoon water
2 tablespoons grated parmesan cheese

Sift flour into bowl, make a well in centre, gradually stir in combined egg, milk and oil; stir until smooth. Stand 30 minutes. Batter can be made in a blender or processor.

Grease a small, heavy-based pan, pour quarter of batter into pan, cook until set; turn, cook other side.

Makes 4 crepes.

Filling: Combine beans, corn, peppers, onion and chilli in a frying pan; cook, stirring, 2 minutes. Add undrained, crushed tomatoes and wine, bring to the boil, reduce heat, simmer, uncovered, for 15 minutes. Stir in blended cornflour and water, stir constantly over heat until mixture boils and thickens (or microwave on HIGH for about 10 minutes).

Place quarter of the filling onto each crepe, roll up. Place in ovenproof dish in single layer, sprinkle with cheese, bake, uncovered, in moderate oven for about 10 minutes (or microwave on HIGH for 4 minutes or until crepes are heated through).

Serves 4.

Approximately 870 kilojoules (208 calories) per serve.

PUMPKIN NESTS

This recipe is not suitable to freeze.

2 x 400g golden nugget pumpkins
1 teaspoon butter
1 small onion (80g), finely chopped
10 spinach (silver beet) leaves (200g), chopped
60g fetta cheese, crumbled
pinch ground nutmeg
1 egg, lightly beaten
1 tablespoon grated tasty cheese

Cut pumpkins in half and remove seeds. Boil, steam or microwave pumpkins until just tender; drain.

Melt butter in saucepan, add onion, cook, stirring, until onion is soft. Add spinach, cover, cook until wilted. Place onion mixture in bowl, add fetta cheese, nutmeg and egg; mix well. Fill each pumpkin half with spinach mixture, top with tasty cheese. Place on oven tray, bake in moderate oven for about 15 minutes (or microwave on HIGH for about 3 minutes).

Serves 4.

Approximately 565 kilojoules (135 calories) per serve.

ABOVE: Pumpkin Nests. LEFT: Top: Zucchini and Avocado Omelet Rolls; bottom: Chilli and Corn Crepes

SQUID WITH TOMATO SAUCE

Squid can be prepared up to 3 hours before required. This recipe is not suitable to freeze or microwave.

4 x 125g baby squid
½ cup rice (100g)
1 tablespoon oil
1 medium onion (120g), chopped
1 clove garlic, crushed
1 tablespoon tomato paste
2 tablespoons currants
2 tablespoons chopped fresh parsley
¼ cup dry white wine
½ cup water
1 tablespoon lemon juice
TOMATO SAUCE
1 clove garlic, crushed
1 small onion (80g), chopped
½ cup water
2 medium ripe tomatoes (200g), peeled and chopped
1 small chicken stock cube, crumbled
1 tablespoon tomato paste

Hold squid firmly with one hand, hold head and pull gently with other hand. Head and inside of body of squid will come away in a complete piece; reserve tentacles. Remove bone which will be found at open end of squid; it looks like a long piece of plastic. Clean squid under cold water, then rub off outer skin; chop tentacles.

Add rice to large saucepan of boiling water, boil, uncovered, for about 12 minutes, or until rice is tender; drain.

Heat oil in frying pan, add onion and garlic, stir constantly over heat until onion is soft, add tentacles, cover, cook few minutes until tentacles are tender. Stir in rice, tomato paste, currants and parsley, mix well; cool to room temperature.

Spoon rice mixture into each squid hood, secure openings with toothpicks. Place squid in a single layer in an ovenproof dish. Add wine, water and lemon juice, cover, bake in moderate oven for 1 hour or until squid are tender. Slice squid, serve with sauce.

Tomato Sauce: Combine garlic, onion and quarter cup of the water in frying pan. Stir constantly over heat until onion is soft. Add tomatoes, stock cube, remaining water and tomato paste. Bring to the boil, reduce heat, simmer, uncovered, for about 5 minutes or until mixture thickens slightly. Blend or process tomato mixture until smooth.

Serves 4.

Approximately 1185 kilojoules (283 calories) per serve.

VINE LEAF PARCELS WITH LEMON SAUCE

If available, fresh vine leaves can be used; they should be blanched first (see Glossary, page 124). Vine leaf parcels can be prepared up to 2 days before required, or frozen for up to 1 month. Sauce is best prepared just before serving. This recipe is not suitable to microwave.

1 teaspoon oil
6 green shallots, chopped
2 tablespoons pine nuts
½ cup rice (100g)
1 tablespoon chopped fresh parsley
2 teaspoons chopped fresh dill
1 teaspoon chopped fresh mint
2 teaspoons lemon juice
1 small chicken stock cube, crumbled
1 cup water
200g packet vine leaves
1 tablespoon lemon juice, extra
LEMON SAUCE
1 egg, separated
2 tablespoons lemon juice
1 small chicken stock cube, crumbled
¾ cup water
2 teaspoons cornflour
1 tablespoon water, extra

Heat oil in saucepan, add shallots, pine nuts and rice; cook, stirring, 3 minutes. Add parsley, dill, mint, lemon juice, stock cube and water. Cover, bring to the boil, reduce heat, simmer 10 minutes or until water is absorbed.

Rinse all the vine leaves under cold water, pat dry with absorbent paper. Place a heaped teaspoon of rice mixture in the centre of 16 vine leaves. Roll up firmly, tucking in ends.

Line base and sides of a saucepan with two thirds of the remaining vine leaves. Place the vine leaf parcels in the saucepan, sprinkle with extra lemon juice, and top with a layer of remaining vine leaves. Place an inverted plate over vine leaves to weigh them down during cooking.

Add enough water to barely cover the plate, cover pan, bring to boil, reduce heat, simmer for 1 hour. Remove pan from heat; stand, covered, for 1 hour. Carefully remove vine leaf parcels from pan, serve with hot sauce.

Lemon Sauce: Whisk egg white in bowl until soft peaks form, gradually whisk in combined egg yolk and lemon juice. Heat stock cube and water in saucepan, stir in blended cornflour and extra water, stir constantly over heat until sauce boils and thickens, cool 5 minutes. Whisk in egg mixture.

Serves 4.

Approximately 735 kilojoules (175 calories) per serve.

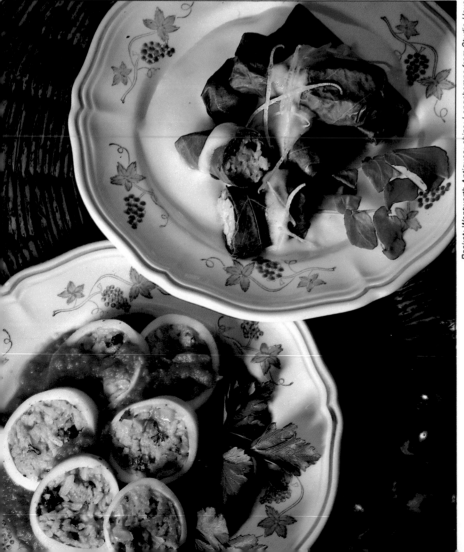

Basket: Wentworth Antiques; china: Longchamps from Studio-Haus

LEFT: Top: Vine Leaf Parcels with Lemon Sauce; bottom: Squid with Tomato Sauce. RIGHT: Clockwise from top: Quick Chicken Surprises; Spinach Ricotta Potatoes; Prawn and Cucumber Cups

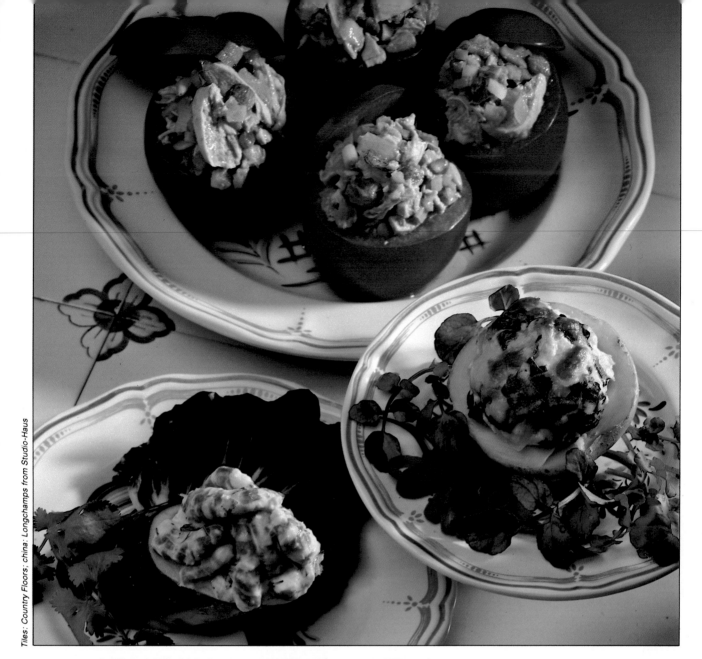

Tiles: Country Floors; china: Longchamps from Studio-Haus

SPINACH RICOTTA POTATOES

Potatoes can be prepared to stage of cooking up to 6 hours ahead. This recipe is not suitable to freeze.

2 large potatoes (370g)
4 spinach (silver beet) leaves (80g)
½ cup ricotta cheese (100g)
¼ teaspoon mixed herbs
2 tablespoons grated mozzarella cheese

Boil, steam or microwave whole potatoes until tender. Cut potatoes in half, scoop out flesh, leaving a half centimetre shell. Remove stalks from spinach. Shred leaves finely; boil, steam or microwave until tender. Combine spinach, ricotta cheese, herbs and chopped potato; fill potato shells with mixture. Top potatoes with mozzarella cheese, bake in moderately hot oven for about 12 minutes (or microwave on HIGH for about 2 minutes).

Serves 4.

Approximately 610 kilojoules (145 calories) per serve.

PRAWN AND CUCUMBER CUPS

This recipe is not suitable to freeze.

250g cooked prawns, shelled
⅓ cup low-fat plain yoghurt
1 small fresh red chilli, finely chopped
2 teaspoons grated fresh ginger
1 clove garlic, crushed
1 teaspoon chopped fresh coriander
2 medium cucumbers (560g)

Combine prawns, yoghurt, chilli, ginger, garlic and coriander in bowl, cover, refrigerate for 1 hour. Make 4 cups by cutting cucumbers diagonally into 5cm slices, scoop out enough seeds to make a hollow in each cup. Fill with prawn mixture.

Serves 4.

Approximately 430 kilojoules (103 calories) per serve.

QUICK CHICKEN SURPRISES

We used barbecued chicken, with the skin removed. This recipe is not suitable to freeze.

1 tablespoon pine nuts
4 medium firm ripe tomatoes (400g), peeled
15g butter
1 small onion (80g), finely chopped
1 clove garlic, crushed
½ cup finely chopped cooked chicken (100g)
1 tablespoon sultanas
3 green shallots, chopped
2 tablespoons low-fat plain yoghurt

Toast pine nuts on oven tray in moderate oven for 5 minutes. Cut tops from tomatoes, scoop out pulp, blend or process pulp until smooth, strain.

Heat butter in a frying pan, add onion and garlic, stir constantly over heat until onion is soft. Stir in pine nuts, chicken, sultanas, shallots, pureed tomato and yoghurt. Fill tomatoes with chicken mixture. Place lids decoratively before serving.

Serves 4.

Approximately 500 kilojoules (120 calories) per serve.

MAIN COURSES

There are around 100 delicious main course recipes in this section, which will probably be the most-used section in the book.
Here are some points which apply to the main courses in general.

■ The weights for individual cuts of meat, chicken and fish, etc., are a guide only; however, these uncooked weights are in line with our kilojoule counter on page 62.

■ Remove any fat from uncooked meat and chicken; always remove skin from chicken.

■ The weights in the recipes are the weights bought from the shops; always buy the leanest meat possible.

■ Try to eat at least one meal a week based on fish. Some low-cholesterol diets may restrict prawns and squid, etc.

■ More vegetarian ideas can be found in the Entrees and Side Dishes sections.

■ Microwave cooking times have been included where we feel they are applicable; cooking times are approximate. Covering the food helps it to cook quicker and stay moist; check your microwave instruction book for further information.

■ The photographs in this section have often had vegetables or rice or similar added to the plate to enhance the appearance of the meal. If the recipe does not contain these vegetables in the list of ingredients, then they have NOT been included in the kilojoule count. You will have to estimate your kilojoule allowance and add accompaniments to suit your requirements.

■ Oil and butter (use your favourite margarine, if you prefer) have been kept to a minimum throughout this book. Sometimes oil and butter can be eliminated from recipes by using a non-stick frying pan or a pan sprayed with one of the readily available non-stick sprays.

■ Always read the labels on canned and packaged foods to discover the salt content; we have not added extra salt to any of the recipes.

■ If you are on a low-salt diet, take extra care to check labels on various products.

■ Make your own salt-free and fat-free stock (see Glossary, page 124) if preferred, instead of stock cubes and water as indicated in recipes.

■ Pepper is used rarely in our recipes; season according to your own taste.

■ Fresh herbs are used freely for their wonderful flavours. Dried, freeze-dried and ground herbs are more concentrated than fresh; see Glossary, page 124, for more information. Experiment with different fresh herbs to create your own sensational taste variations.

■ If you would like to serve these recipes to the rest of your non-dieting family, simply add more meat, fish or chicken, and hearty servings of vegetables or salad, or bread, rice or pasta.

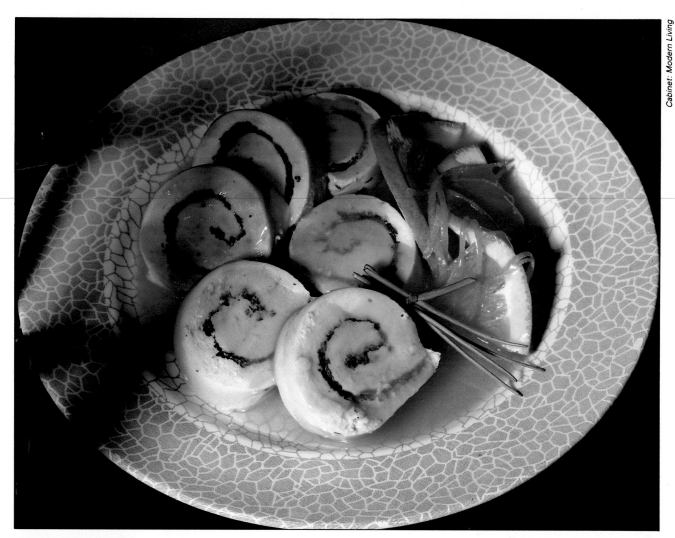

Cabinet: Modern Living

MAIN COURSES
CHICKEN

Chicken is a dieter's dream because it has such good flavour, is easy to prepare and cooks quickly. Always remove the skin from the chicken as it is very fatty; also remove any visible fat. If you have bought chicken on the bone, use the bones and any bits and pieces of chicken to make stock, see Glossary on page 124.

MINTED CHICKEN WITH SWEET ORANGE SAUCE

This recipe is not suitable to freeze or microwave.

4 x 115g chicken breast fillets
¾ cup chopped fresh mint
SWEET ORANGE SAUCE
½ cup white vinegar
1 tablespoon sugar
1 cup strained orange juice
1 teaspoon cornflour
1 teaspoon water
1 teaspoon butter

Flatten the chicken evenly with a meat mallet. Spread mint evenly over each chicken fillet, roll up tightly, secure with toothpicks. Place in ovenproof dish in a single layer, bake, covered, in moderate oven for 25 minutes, or until chicken is tender. Remove toothpicks, slice chicken, serve with sauce.

Sweet Orange Sauce: Combine vinegar and sugar in small saucepan, stir constantly over heat, without boiling, until sugar is dissolved. Bring to the boil, boil rapidly, without stirring, until mixture turns light golden brown. Add orange juice, bring to the boil, reduce heat, simmer mixture, uncovered, until reduced by half. Add blended cornflour and water, stir constantly over heat until sauce boils and thickens. Whisk in butter just before serving.

Serves 4.

Approximately 790 kilojoules (188 calories) per serve.

Minted Chicken with Sweet Orange Sauce

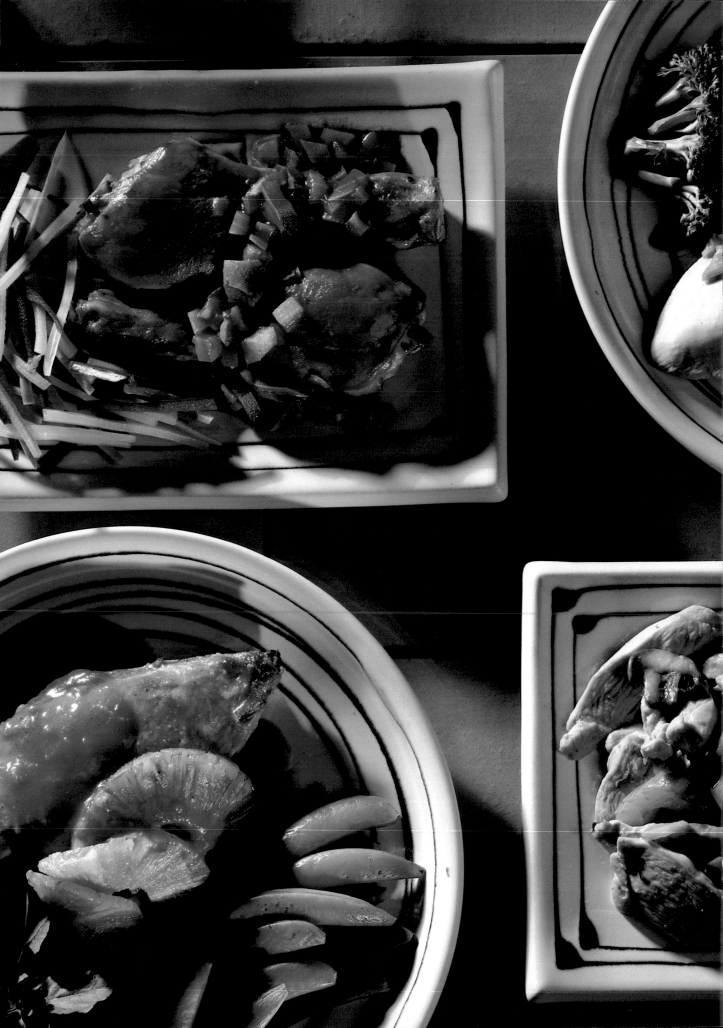

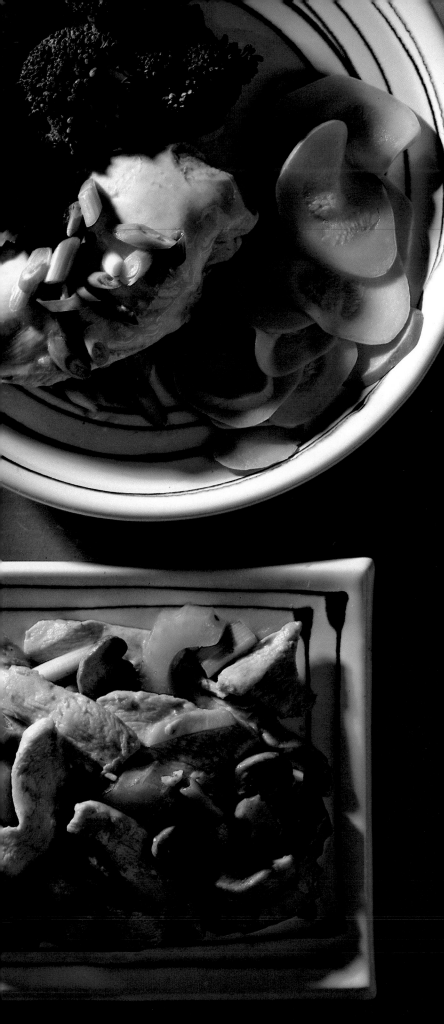

CHILLI CHICKEN

This recipe can be made up to 2 days ahead; it is not suitable to freeze.

8 x 85g chicken drumsticks
1 small fresh red chilli, chopped
2 tablespoons oyster sauce
1 clove garlic, crushed
TOMATO SAUCE
½ cup tomato purée
1 small stick celery (60g), chopped
1 medium onion (120g), chopped
1 medium green pepper (150g),
    chopped
1 teaspoon sesame oil

Combine chicken, chilli, oyster sauce and garlic in a large bowl, mix well. Place chicken in single layer in baking dish. Bake in moderate oven for about 30 minutes (or microwave on HIGH for about 10 minutes) or until chicken is tender, turn once during cooking, serve with sauce.

Tomato Sauce: Combine tomato purée, celery, onion, pepper and sesame oil in a small saucepan. Bring to the boil, reduce heat, simmer, uncovered, for about 5 minutes or until sauce is slightly thickened (or microwave on HIGH for about 5 minutes).

Serves 4.

Approximately 940 kilojoules (224 calories) per serve.

LEMON SHALLOT CHICKEN

This recipe is unsuitable to freeze.

1 small chicken stock cube,
    crumbled
1 cup water
1 clove garlic, crushed
4 x 115g chicken breast fillets
1½ tablespoons lemon juice
6 green shallots, finely chopped

Combine stock cube, water and garlic in frying pan, bring to the boil, add chicken, reduce heat, simmer until just tender (or microwave on HIGH for about 6 minutes). Remove chicken from pan.

Add lemon juice to pan, boil until mixture is reduced by half (or microwave on HIGH for about 3 minutes), stir in shallots, serve over chicken.

Serves 4.

Approximately 565 kilojoules (135 calories) per serve.

China: Made in Japan

*Clockwise from top left: Chilli Chicken;
Lemon Shallot Chicken; Stir-Fried
Chicken with Water Chestnuts; Curried
Pineapple Chicken*

CURRIED PINEAPPLE CHICKEN

Recipe unsuitable to freeze.

440g can unsweetened sliced pineapple
2 tablespoons light soya sauce
1 teaspoon curry powder
1 clove garlic, crushed
1 teaspoon grated fresh ginger
4 x 200g chicken breasts on the bone
1 teaspoon cornflour

Drain pineapple, reserve juice. Combine pineapple juice, soya sauce, curry powder, garlic and ginger in bowl, add chicken, mix well, cover, refrigerate several hours or overnight.

Place chicken on a wire rack over baking dish, bake in moderate oven for about 30 minutes (or microwave on HIGH for about 12 minutes) or until chicken is tender, brush occasionally with about half the marinade during cooking time.

Cut pineapple rings in half, top chicken with pineapple. Return chicken to oven for further 5 minutes (or microwave on HIGH 30 seconds). Blend cornflour with remaining marinade in saucepan, stir constantly over heat until mixture boils and thickens (or microwave on HIGH 1 minute). Serve sauce over chicken.

Serves 4.

Approximately 995 kilojoules (238 calories) per serve.

STIR-FRIED CHICKEN WITH WATER CHESTNUTS

This recipe is not suitable to freeze or microwave.

3 x 115g chicken breast fillets
2 tablespoons light soya sauce
2 teaspoons oil
1 clove garlic, crushed
1 teaspoon finely chopped fresh ginger
1 large stick celery (100g), sliced
40g mushrooms, sliced
⅓ cup canned water chestnuts (50g), sliced
2 green shallots, chopped
2 teaspoons cornflour
1 tablespoon dry sherry
¼ cup water

Cut chicken into thin strips, marinate in bowl with half the soya sauce.

Heat oil in wok or frying pan, add garlic and ginger, add chicken, stir-fry until chicken is tender. Add celery, mushrooms, water chestnuts and shallots, stir-fry 1 minute. Blend cornflour with remaining soya sauce, sherry and water, add to chicken mixture, stir constantly over heat until the mixture boils and thickens.

Serves 4.

Approximately 560 kilojoules (133 calories) per serve.

MUSTARD CHIVE CHICKEN

Recipe unsuitable to freeze.

4 x 115g chicken breast fillets
2 teaspoons French mustard
2 teaspoons oil
½ cup water
1 small chicken stock cube, crumbled
2 teaspoons cornflour
2 tablespoons water, extra
⅓ cup evaporated skim milk
2 tablespoons chopped fresh chives

Spread chicken with mustard. Heat oil in a frying pan, add chicken and cook until browned.

Stir in water and stock cube, simmer, uncovered, 10 minutes (or microwave on HIGH for about 6 minutes) or until tender. Blend cornflour with extra water, add to chicken mixture, stir constantly over heat until mixture boils and thickens (or microwave on HIGH for about 1 minute). Stir in milk and chives, reheat before serving.

Serves 4.

Approximately 735 kilojoules (175 calories) per serve.

APRICOT GINGER CHICKEN

This recipe is not suitable to freeze or microwave.

4 x 115g chicken breast fillets
1 tablespoon oil
APRICOT SAUCE
2cm piece fresh ginger, peeled
¾ cup apricot nectar
2 teaspoons dry sherry
1 teaspoon light soya sauce
1 teaspoon cornflour
2 teaspoons water
1 green shallot, chopped
¼ teaspoon ground cumin

Cut each fillet into strips. Heat oil in frying pan, add chicken, cook, stirring, until golden brown. Remove from pan, place onto serving dish with sauce.

Apricot Sauce: Cut ginger into wafer-thin slices, then into shreds, combine in saucepan with apricot nectar, sherry and soya sauce, bring to the boil, stir in blended cornflour and water, stir constantly over heat until sauce boils and thickens, add shallot and cumin.

Serves 4.

Approximately 870 kilojoules (208 calories) per serve.

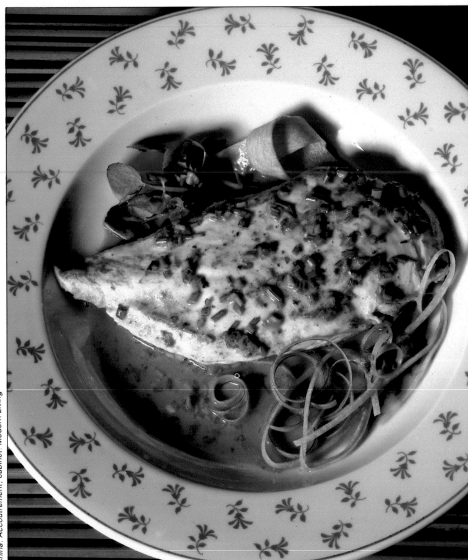

Tiles: Pazotti; china: Made in Japan

China: Accoutrement; cabinet: Modern Living

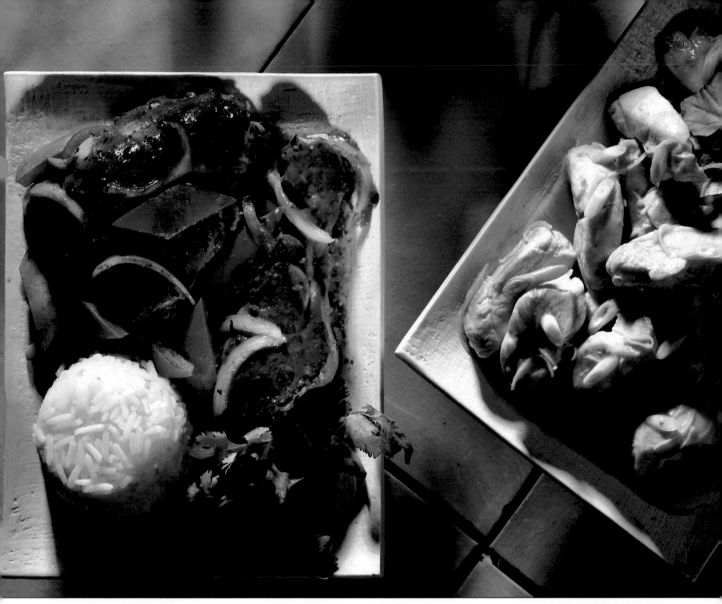

CHICKEN IN BLACK BEAN SAUCE WITH PEPPERS

Black beans are an imported product available from most supermarkets and Asian food stores. You will need to cook one-third cup rice for this recipe. This recipe is unsuitable to freeze.

4 x 375g chicken marylands
2 tablespoons canned black beans, rinsed, drained, mashed
2 tablespoons light soya sauce
1 tablespoon dry sherry
2 cloves garlic, crushed
2 teaspoons grated fresh ginger
2 tablespoons water
1 medium green pepper (150g), chopped
1 medium red pepper (150g), chopped
1 medium onion (120g), sliced
2 teaspoons cornflour
¼ cup water, extra
1 cup cooked rice

Cut marylands at the joint into 2 pieces. Combine chicken in bowl with black beans, soya sauce, sherry, garlic and ginger, marinate for 1 hour or refrigerate, covered, overnight.

Heat water in a large frying pan, place chicken mixture into pan, cook, turning often, for about 15 minutes, or until chicken is tender (or microwave on HIGH for about 7 minutes). Add peppers and onion, stir constantly over heat for about 2 minutes (or microwave on HIGH for about 2 minutes). Stir in blended cornflour and extra water, stir constantly over heat until mixture boils and thickens (or microwave on HIGH for about 1 minute). Serve with rice.
Serves 4.

Approximately 1190 kilojoules (284 calories) per serve.

CHICKEN PIQUANT

Make this recipe a day ahead to allow most flavour to develop; it can be frozen for up to 2 months.

1 small onion (80g), finely chopped
4 x 75g chicken thigh fillets
1 clove garlic, crushed
2 tablespoons chopped fresh basil
1 medium tomato (100g), peeled, chopped
1 tablespoon tomato paste
1 small chicken stock cube, crumbled
½ cup water
1 small stick celery (60g), sliced
1 small red pepper (100g), sliced
½ medium carrot (60g), sliced
2 teaspoons cornflour
2 tablespoons water, extra

Combine onion and chicken in an ovenproof dish, stir in garlic, basil, tomato, tomato paste, stock cube, water, celery, pepper and carrot; cover, bake in moderate oven 30 minutes (or microwave on HIGH about 10 minutes) or until chicken is tender. Stir in blended cornflour and extra water; bake further 10 minutes or until mixture boils and thickens (or microwave on HIGH about 5 minutes).
Serves 4.

Approximately 525 kilojoules (125 calories) per serve.

ABOVE: Left: Chicken in Black Bean Sauce with Peppers; right: Apricot Ginger Chicken. OPPOSITE PAGE: Mustard Chive Chicken

27

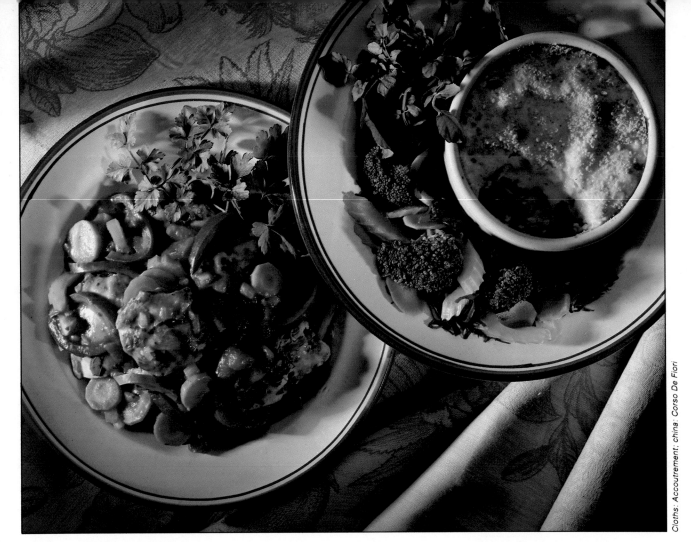

Cloths: Accoutrement; china: Corso De Fiori

SAUCY CHICKEN CASSEROLES

This recipe is not suitable to freeze or microwave.

115g chicken breast fillet
2 teaspoons oil
1 medium onion (120g), finely chopped
1 clove garlic, crushed
425g can tomatoes
¼ teaspoon dried basil leaves
¼ teaspoon dried oregano leaves
¼ teaspoon sugar
1 tablespoon grated parmesan cheese
1 tablespoon packaged breadcrumbs
TOPPING
15g butter
1 tablespoon plain flour
¾ cup skim milk
¼ teaspoon dry mustard
1 egg, lightly beaten

Poach, steam or microwave chicken until just tender, chop chicken.

Heat oil in saucepan, add onion and garlic, stir constantly over heat until onion is soft. Stir in undrained, crushed tomatoes, herbs and sugar, bring to the boil, reduce heat, simmer, uncovered, 10 minutes or until mixture is thick; stir in chicken.

Divide mixture into 4 ovenproof dishes (three-quarter cup capacity), spread evenly with topping. Sprinkle with combined cheese and breadcrumbs. Bake in moderate oven for about 20 minutes or until cheese is lightly browned.

Topping: Melt butter in saucepan, stir in flour, stir constantly over heat for 1 minute. Gradually stir in milk, stir constantly over heat until mixture boils and thickens. Remove from heat, stir in mustard and egg.

Serves 4.

Approximately 1095 kilojoules (262 calories) per serve.

SPICY CHICKEN TACOS

Follow packet directions for heating taco shells. This recipe is not suitable to freeze or microwave.

115g chicken breast fillet
1 medium onion (120g), finely chopped
1 clove garlic, crushed
1 tablespoon water
425g can tomatoes
1 canned jalapeno chilli, finely chopped
½ cup canned red kidney beans, rinsed, drained
1 cup shredded lettuce (60g)
4 taco shells
½ cup grated tasty cheese (60g)

Poach, steam, microwave or grill chicken until tender; cool, chop finely.

Combine onion, garlic and water in frying pan, stir constantly over heat until onion is soft (or microwave on HIGH for about 3 minutes). Stir in undrained, crushed tomatoes and chilli, bring to the boil, reduce heat, simmer until almost all the liquid is absorbed, stir occasionally. Stir in chicken and half the beans, then stir in remaining mashed beans, reheat, stirring constantly. Place lettuce in hot taco shells, top with chicken mixture, then cheese.

Serves 4.

Approximately 1210 kilojoules (290 calories) per serve.

ABOVE: From left: Chicken Piquant; Saucy Chicken Casseroles. Right: Spicy Chicken Tacos

Tray & china: Accoutrement

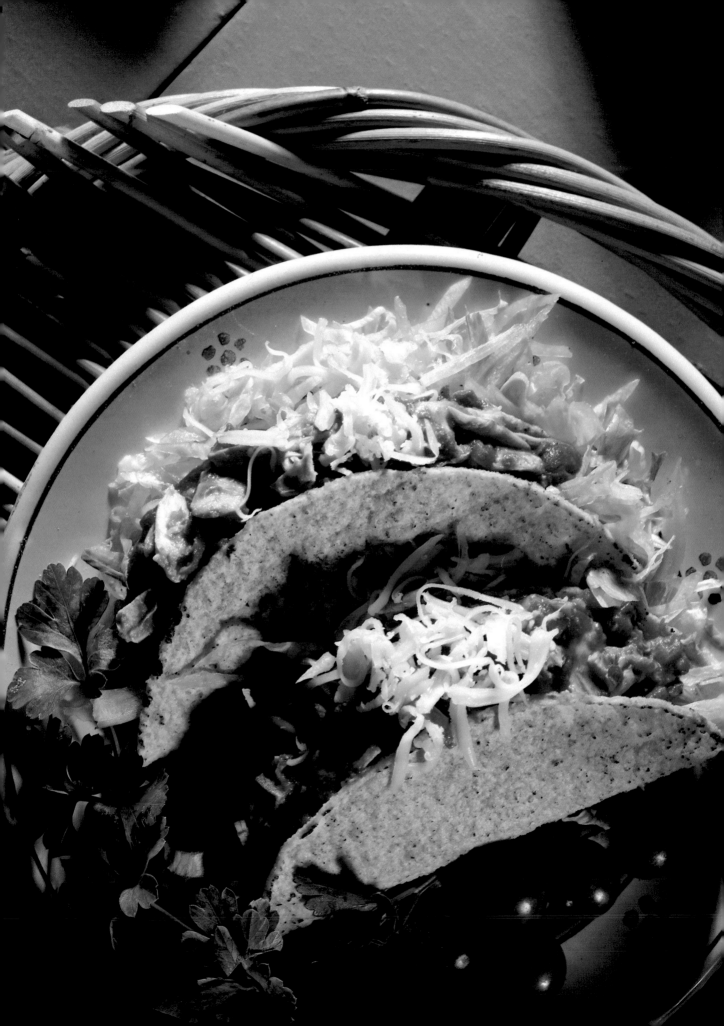

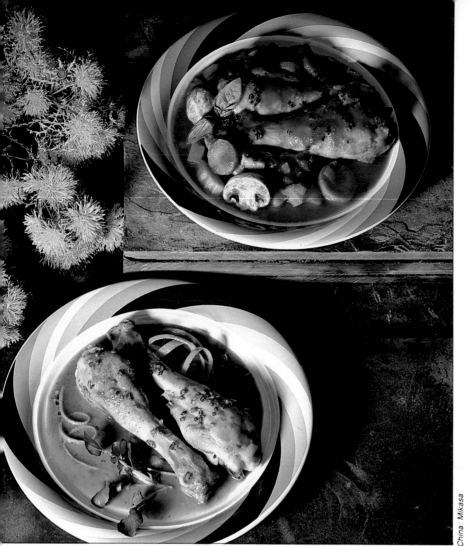

CREAMY ASPARAGUS CHICKEN WITH PEPPERCORNS

Recipe unsuitable to freeze.

4 x 115g chicken breast fillets
1 tablespoon dry vermouth
½ cup water
1 small chicken stock cube,
 crumbled
340g can asparagus spears
1 medium onion (120g), finely
 chopped
2 teaspoons drained canned green
 peppercorns
2 teaspoons seeded mustard
1 tablespoon chopped fresh parsley
2 tablespoons sour light cream
2 teaspoons cornflour
1 tablespoon water, extra

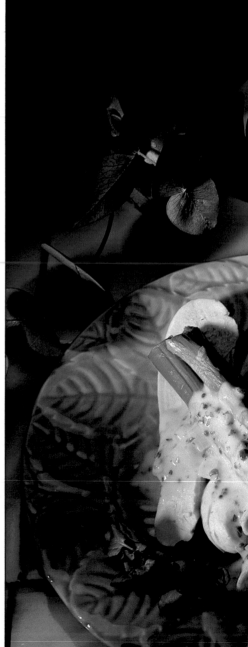

China: Mikasa

CHICKEN DRUMSTICK CASSEROLE WITH MUSHROOMS

This recipe is not suitable to freeze or microwave.

2 teaspoons oil
8 x 85g chicken drumsticks
2 medium sticks celery (160g),
 chopped
1 large carrot (200g), sliced
1 medium onion (120g), chopped
425g can tomatoes
1 small chicken stock cube,
 crumbled
1 tablespoon cornflour
½ cup water
90g baby mushrooms, halved
1 tablespoon chopped fresh parsley
Heat oil in frying pan, add chicken, cook until lightly browned, remove from pan, drain on absorbent paper.

Add celery, carrot and onion to pan, stir over heat for 1 minute. Add undrained, crushed tomatoes and stock cube, bring to the boil. Stir in blended cornflour and water, stir constantly over heat until mixture boils and thickens. Add chicken and mushrooms, cover, simmer 15 minutes or until chicken is tender. Sprinkle with parsley just before serving.
 Serves 4.

Approximately 1030 kilojoules (246 calories) per serve.

SHERRIED CHICKEN

This dish can be frozen for up to 2 months; add chives just before serving the dish.

2 teaspoons oil
8 x 85g chicken drumsticks
1 small chicken stock cube,
 crumbled
1 cup water
¼ cup dry sherry
2 tablespoons chopped fresh chives
Heat oil in frying pan, add chicken, cook until lightly browned. Stir in stock cube and water, bring to the boil, reduce heat, simmer, covered, for about 20 minutes, or until chicken is tender (or microwave on HIGH for about 10 minutes). Remove chicken from pan, add sherry to pan, boil until reduced by half. Return chicken to pan, reheat. Serve sprinkled with chives.
 Serves 4.

Approximately 835 kilojoules (199 calories) per serve.

Place chicken in frying pan, add vermouth, water and stock cube. Drain asparagus, reserve liquid, add liquid to pan with chicken, bring to the boil, reduce heat, cover, simmer 10 minutes, or until chicken is tender (or microwave on HIGH for about 5 minutes). Remove chicken from pan; slice and keep warm.

Add onion to liquid in pan, simmer few minutes, or until onion is soft. Stir in crushed peppercorns, mustard, parsley and cream. Blend cornflour with extra water, add to pan, stir constantly over heat until mixture boils and thickens (or microwave on HIGH for about 3 minutes). Serve over chicken topped with asparagus spears.

Serves 4.

Approximately 760 kilojoules (182 calories) per serve.

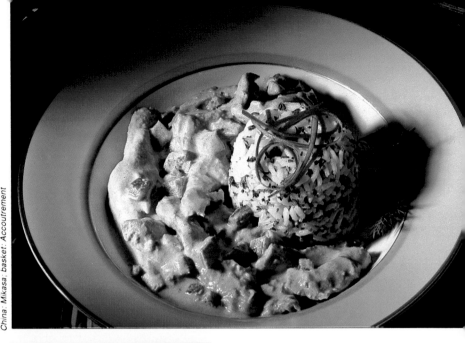

China: Mikasa; basket: Accoutrement

CHICKEN AND CHEESE WITH LEMON SAUCE

Recipe unsuitable to freeze.

4 x 115g chicken breast fillets
¼ cup cottage cheese (60g)
2 teaspoons chopped fresh chives
¼ teaspoon dried tarragon leaves
1 small chicken stock cube, crumbled
1 cup water
LEMON SAUCE
2 teaspoons cornflour
½ cup water
2 tablespoons lemon juice
2 teaspoons sugar
2 teaspoons butter

Cut a pocket in the thickest part of each fillet. Combine sieved cottage cheese, chives and tarragon in a bowl; mix well. Fill pockets with cottage cheese mixture. Place chicken in an ovenproof dish with combined stock cube and water, cover, bake in moderate oven for about 20 minutes (or microwave on HIGH for about 5 minutes) or until tender. Remove chicken from stock, serve topped with sauce.

Lemon Sauce: Blend cornflour with water in a small saucepan, add lemon juice and sugar. Stir constantly over heat until mixture boils and thickens (or microwave on HIGH for about 3 minutes); stir in butter.

Serves 4.

Approximately 740 kilojoules (177 calories) per serve.

China & napkin: Accoutrement; tiles: Country Floors

LEFT: Top: Chicken and Cheese with Lemon Sauce; bottom: Creamy Asparagus Chicken with Peppercorns. FAR LEFT: Top: Chicken Drumstick Casserole with Mushrooms; bottom: Sherried Chicken. ABOVE: Creamy Chicken Paprika

CREAMY CHICKEN PAPRIKA

This recipe is unsuitable to freeze.

4 x 115g chicken breast fillets
½ cup sour light cream
1 small chicken stock cube,
**   crumbled**
2 tablespoons water
1 teaspoon paprika
1 tablespoon tomato paste
1 medium red pepper (150g),
**   chopped**
1 medium green pepper (150g),
**   chopped**

Cut chicken into strips. Combine cream, stock cube, water, paprika and tomato paste in a large saucepan, bring to the boil. Stir in chicken and peppers, reduce heat, simmer, uncovered, for about 3 minutes or until the chicken is tender (or microwave on HIGH for about 5 minutes).

Serves 4.

Approximately 860 kilojoules (205 calories) per serve.

CHICKEN AND VEGERONI BAKE

Vegeroni is a pasta based on several types of vegetables. You will need to cook half cup vegeroni for this recipe; the dish is unsuitable to freeze.

115g chicken breast fillet
15g butter
4 green shallots, finely chopped
125g mushrooms, sliced
2 tablespoons plain flour
1 cup skim milk
½ cup water
1 small chicken stock cube,
**   crumbled**
1 cup cooked vegeroni
¼ cup stale breadcrumbs
2 tablespoons grated parmesan
**   cheese**
2 teaspoons chopped fresh parsley

Poach, steam, microwave or grill chicken until tender; cool, chop roughly.

Melt butter in saucepan, add shallots and mushrooms, stir constantly over heat until mushrooms are soft, stir in flour, stir over heat for 1 minute. Gradually stir in milk, water and stock cube, stir constantly over heat until mixture boils and thickens (or microwave on HIGH for about 5 minutes). Remove the mixture from heat, stir in chicken and vegeroni.

Spoon mixture into 4 ovenproof dishes (three-quarter cup capacity), top with combined breadcrumbs, cheese and parsley. Bake in moderate oven for about 15 minutes or until browned (or microwave on HIGH for about 3 minutes).

Serves 4.

Approximately 1140 kilojoules (272 calories) per serve.

MARINATED CHICKEN KEBABS

Soak 12 bamboo skewers in water for at least an hour so they won't burn during cooking. This recipe is not suitable to freeze.

4 x 115g chicken breast fillets
2 tablespoons light soya sauce
2 teaspoons oil
1 clove garlic, crushed
1 teaspoon grated fresh ginger
12 small mushrooms (225g), halved
12 cherry tomatoes (70g)
1 small green pepper (100g),
**   chopped**
4 x 50g slices fresh pineapple,
**   chopped**

Cut chicken into 2cm pieces, combine in bowl with soya sauce, oil, garlic and ginger; marinate 1 hour, or refrigerate chicken in mixture overnight.

Thread chicken, mushrooms, tomatoes, pepper and pineapple onto skewers. Grill gently, basting frequently with marinade, on both sides until tender (or microwave on HIGH for about 3 minutes).

Serves 4.

Approximately 800 kilojoules (190 calories) per serve.

BELOW: Chicken and Vegeroni Bake.
RIGHT: Marinated Chicken Kebabs

Tea-towel & tray: The Design Store; china: Sasaki from Dansab

Dish: Accoutrement; cabinet & placemat: Modern Living

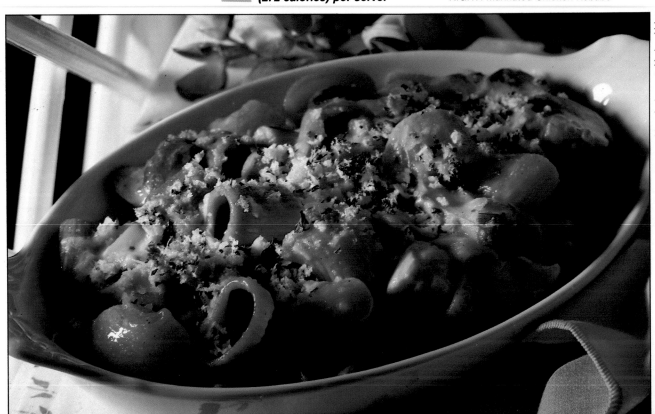

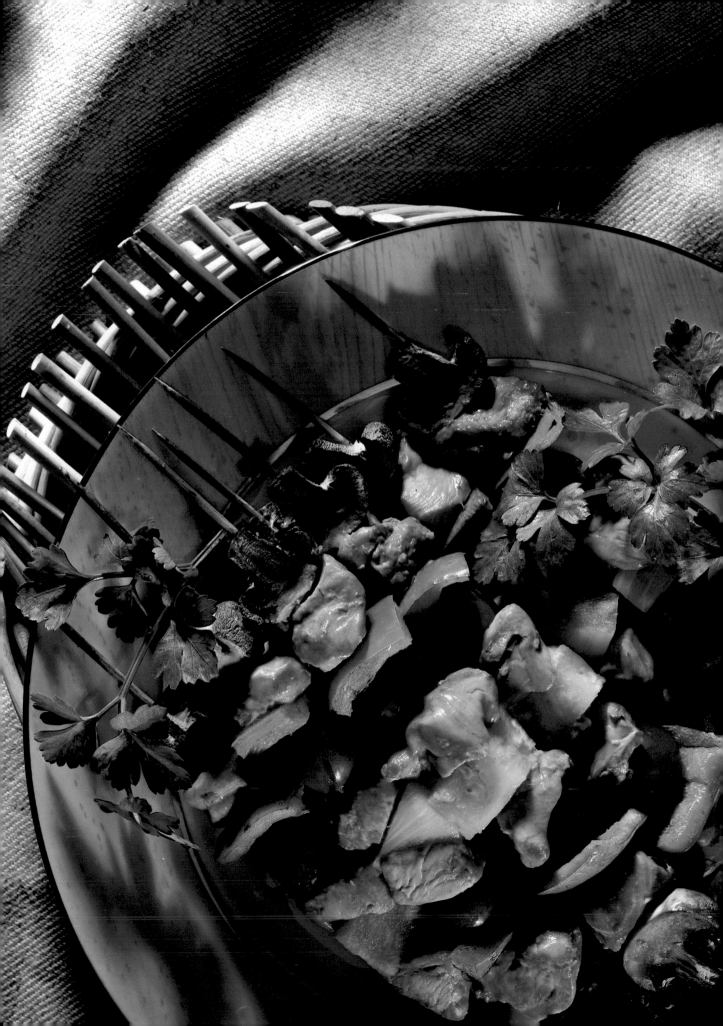

MAIN COURSES
BEEF

We are fortunate to have access to some of the best and leanest beef in the world and it should be included in your diet, particularly as it is a rich source of iron. Any visible fat should be cut away before cooking. If using mince, either mince or process meat you have bought yourself (topside is ideal) or ask the butcher to prepare it.

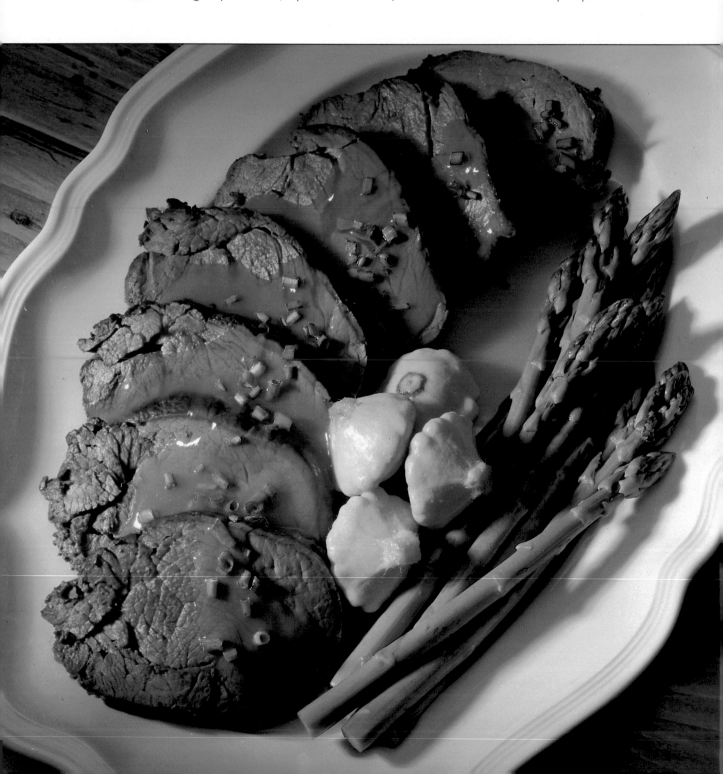

PORT AND GARLIC BEEF

Recipe unsuitable to microwave.

1 tablespoon port
2 teaspoons dark soya sauce
½ teaspoon oil
1 clove garlic, crushed
500g beef eye fillet, in one piece
SAUCE
1 cup water
1 small chicken stock cube, crumbled
1 teaspoon sugar
1 teaspoon tomato paste
1 tablespoon lemon juice
1 tablespoon cornflour
1 tablespoon water
1 tablespoon chopped fresh chives

Combine port, soya sauce, oil and garlic in bowl, add beef. Turn beef, coating well with marinade, cover, refrigerate overnight. Remove beef from marinade, reserve marinade. Tie beef with string to keep in good shape. Place beef in baking dish, bake in moderately hot oven for about 40 minutes or until beef is done as desired. Stand beef 5 minutes before cutting and serve with the sauce.

Sauce: Combine water, stock cube, sugar, tomato paste, lemon juice and reserved marinade in saucepan. Blend cornflour with water, stir into sauce mixture, stir constantly over heat until sauce boils and thickens. Add chives just before serving.

Serves 4.

 Approximately 1040 kilojoules (248 calories) per serve.

CREAMY PEPPERCORN STEAKS

This recipe is not suitable to freeze or microwave.

2 teaspoons oil
4 x 125g lean beef eye fillet steaks
1 medium onion (120g), finely chopped
1 teaspoon canned drained green peppercorns, crushed
2 teaspoons French mustard
1 tablespoon brandy
2 tablespoons water
2 tablespoons sour light cream

Heat oil in frying pan, add steaks, cook until done as desired. Remove steaks from pan, keep steaks warm. Add onion and peppercorns to pan, stir constantly over heat until onion is soft. Stir in mustard, brandy and water, bring to the boil, stir in cream. Return steaks to pan, heat few minutes without boiling.

Serves 4.

 Approximately 870 kilojoules (208 calories) per serve.

BEEF CURRY WITH CRISPY PASTRY PUFFS

Curry can be frozen up to 2 months. Recipe unsuitable to microwave.

2 teaspoons oil
1 small onion (80g), chopped
300g lean minced beef
2 cloves garlic, crushed
1 tablespoon plain flour
2 teaspoons curry powder
1 small chicken stock cube, crumbled
2 cups water
1 tablespoon tomato paste
1 large Granny Smith apple (200g), sliced
1 small potato (75g), sliced
PASTRY PUFFS
⅓ sheet ready-rolled puff pastry

Heat oil in a frying pan, add onion, stir constantly over heat until onion is lightly browned. Add mince and garlic, stir over high heat until well browned. Add flour and curry powder, stir over heat 1 minute. Add stock cube, water and tomato paste, stir constantly over heat until mixture boils and thickens. Add apple and potato, reduce heat, simmer, covered, for 15 minutes or until potato is tender. Serve with pastry puffs.

Pastry Puffs: Cut pastry sheet into 8 squares. Place squares onto oven tray, bake in hot oven for 10 minutes or until golden brown.

Serves 4.

 Approximately 1235 kilojoules (295 calories) per serve.

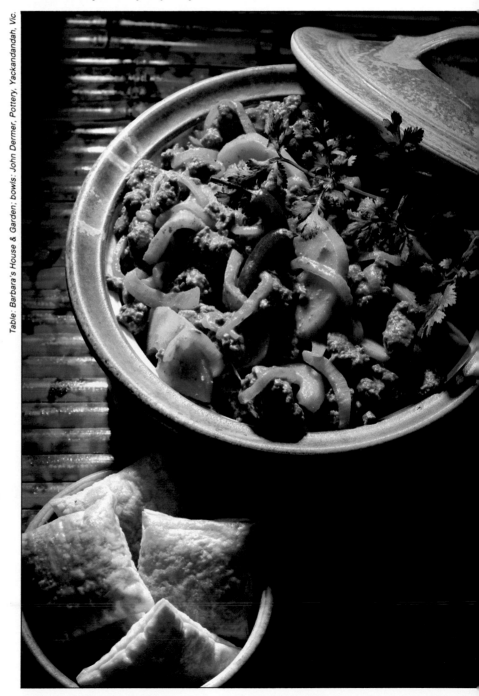

LEFT: Port and Garlic Beef. RIGHT: Beef Curry with Crispy Pastry Puffs

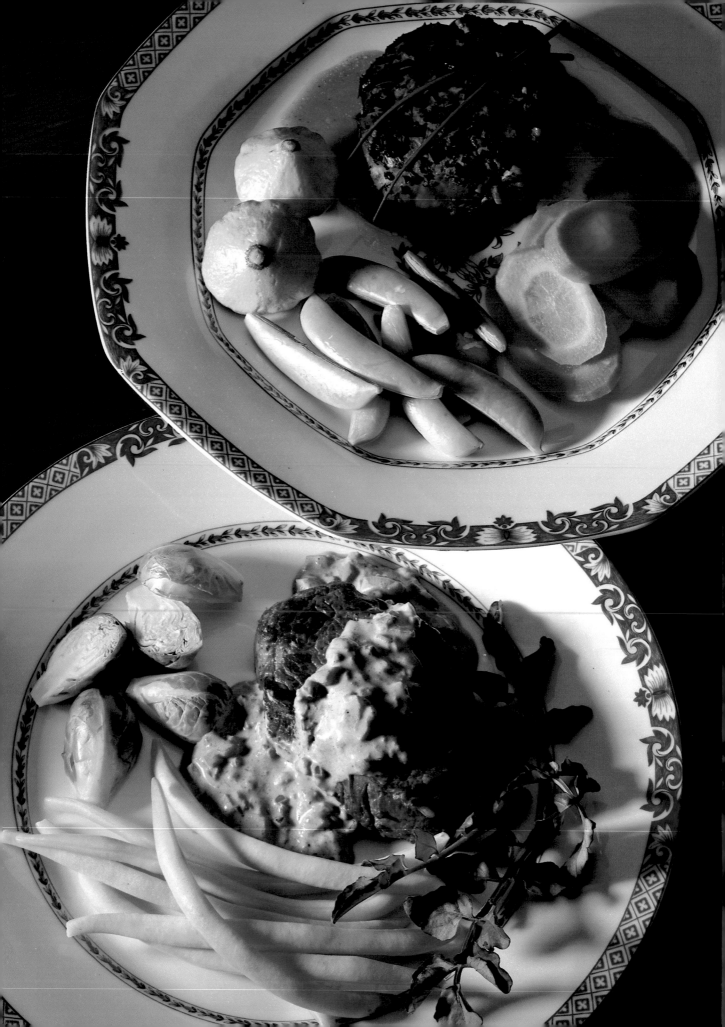

MEATBALLS IN RICH MUSHROOM SAUCE

The meatballs can be frozen for up to 2 months, but the sauce is not suitable to freeze. This recipe is not suitable to microwave.

300g minced steak
1 medium onion (120g), finely chopped
1 clove garlic, crushed
1 tablespoon tomato sauce
1 tablespoon dark soya sauce
½ cup stale breadcrumbs
2 teaspoons oil
RICH MUSHROOM SAUCE
1 bacon rasher (40g), finely chopped
250g mushrooms, thinly sliced
2 teaspoons cornflour
⅔ cup water
1 small beef stock cube, crumbled
¼ teaspoon dried basil leaves

Combine mince, onion, garlic, sauces and breadcrumbs in bowl. Shape tablespoonfuls of mixture into balls, place on tray in single layer, refrigerate 30 minutes.

Heat oil in frying pan, add meatballs, cook gently until well browned all over and cooked through. Remove meatballs from pan and keep warm while making sauce.

Rich Mushroom Sauce: Add bacon and mushrooms to pan in which meatballs were cooked, stir constantly over heat until mushrooms are tender. Stir in blended cornflour and water, stock cube and basil, stir constantly over heat until sauce boils and thickens.

Add meatballs to sauce, simmer, uncovered, until heated through.

Serves 4.

 Approximately 1165 kilojoules (278 calories) per serve.

STEAKS WITH FRESH HERBS

For a stronger flavour, the steaks may be coated in herbs several hours before cooking. This recipe is not suitable to freeze or microwave.

1 clove garlic, crushed
2 tablespoons chopped fresh chives
2 tablespoons chopped fresh parsley
2 tablespoons chopped fresh basil
4 x 125g lean beef eye fillet steaks
2 teaspoons oil
1 cup water
1 small beef stock cube, crumbled
1 teaspoon cornflour
¼ cup water, extra

Combine garlic, chives, parsley and basil, spread over steaks, stand several hours, if desired.

Heat oil in a frying pan, add steaks and cook until done as desired. Remove steaks from pan, keep steaks warm. Add water, stock cube and blended cornflour and extra water to pan, stir constantly over heat until sauce boils and thickens; serve steaks with sauce.

Serves 4.

 Approximately 775 kilojoules (185 calories) per serve.

LEFT: Top: Steaks with Fresh Herbs; bottom: Creamy Peppercorn Steaks.

LIGHT AND TASTY BEEF STROGANOFF

You will need to cook about 100g fettucine for this recipe. This recipe is not suitable to freeze or microwave. It is easy to slice beef if it is partly frozen.

200g lean beef eye fillet
1 tablespoon Worcestershire sauce
2 teaspoons oil
1 clove garlic, crushed
1 medium onion (120g), chopped
200g mushrooms, sliced
2 teaspoons cornflour
1 cup skim milk
1 tablespoon tomato paste
1 small beef stock cube, crumbled
2 cups cooked fettucine
1 tablespoon chopped fresh parsley

Cut beef into wafer thin strips. Place in bowl with sauce, stand 10 minutes.

Heat oil in frying pan, add garlic and beef, stir-fry for about 3 minutes, or until lightly browned all over. Add onion and mushrooms to pan, stir constantly further 2 minutes. Blend cornflour with a little of the milk, add to pan with remaining milk, tomato paste and stock cube; stir constantly over heat until mixture boils and thickens. Reduce heat, simmer, uncovered, 2 minutes. Serve over combined fettucine and parsley.

Serves 4.

 Approximately 1005 kilojoules (240 calories) per serve.

BELOW: Left: Light and Tasty Beef Stroganoff; right: Meatballs in Rich Mushroom Sauce

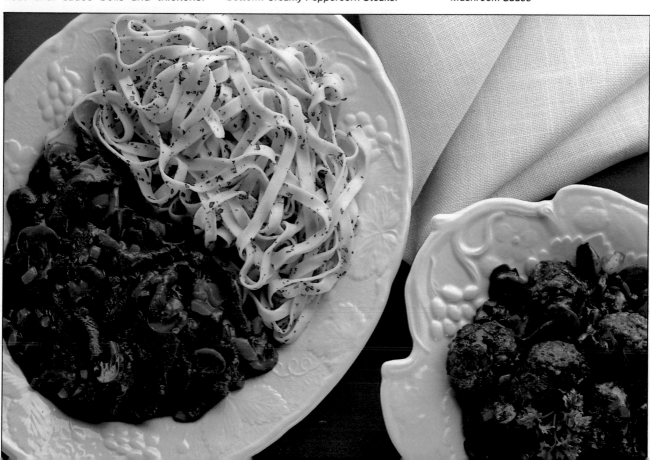

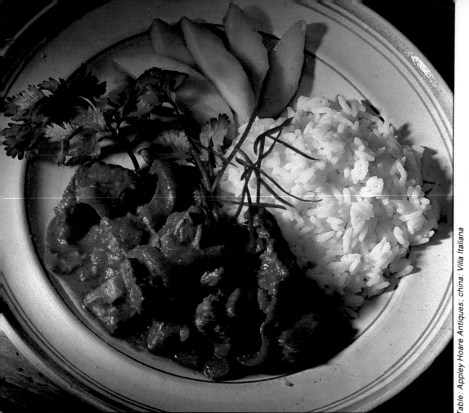

EASY BEEF CURRY

It is best to prepare curry a day before required to allow the flavour to develop. Curry can be frozen for up to 4 months.

400g rump steak
2 medium onions (240g), sliced
1 clove garlic, crushed
1 teaspoon grated fresh ginger
2 teaspoons brown vinegar
2 teaspoons light soya sauce
¼ teaspoon chilli powder
2 teaspoons curry powder
1 tablespoon tomato paste
1 cup water
1 small beef stock cube, crumbled
2 teaspoons cornflour
2 tablespoons water, extra

Cut steak into cubes. Combine steak, onions, garlic, ginger, vinegar, soya sauce, chilli and curry powders, tomato paste, water and stock cube in saucepan. Bring to the boil, reduce heat, simmer, uncovered, 45 minutes, or until steak is tender (or microwave on HIGH for about 15 minutes). Blend cornflour with extra water, add to curry, stir constantly over heat until mixture boils and thickens (or microwave on HIGH for about 3 minutes).

Serves 4.

Approximately 1045 kilojoules (250 calories) per serve.

MEATLOAF WITH BASIL SAUCE

Both meatloaf and sauce can be made a day before required, or frozen for up to 3 months.

300g lean minced beef
1 medium onion (120g), finely chopped
2 teaspoons water
½ cup stale breadcrumbs
1 clove garlic, crushed
2 teaspoons Worcestershire sauce
1 tablespoon light soya sauce
2 tablespoons tomato paste
½ teaspoon dried oregano leaves
1 egg, lightly beaten
BASIL SAUCE
425g can tomatoes
1 clove garlic, crushed
1 tablespoon chopped fresh basil
1 tablespoon tomato paste
1 cup water
1 small beef stock cube, crumbled
1 medium red pepper (150g), sliced

Place mince in bowl. Cook onion with water in a frying pan until onion begins to brown, add to bowl with mince, breadcrumbs, garlic, sauces, tomato paste, oregano and egg; mix well. Press mixture into loaf shape, place into a baking dish, bake, uncovered, in moderate oven for about 40 minutes (or microwave on HIGH for about 10 minutes). Stand 5 minutes before slicing, serve with sauce.

Basil Sauce: Place undrained, crushed tomatoes in saucepan with the remaining ingredients, bring to the boil, reduce heat, simmer, covered, for 30 minutes (or microwave on HIGH for about 15 minutes).

Serves 4.

Approximately 1080 kilojoules (258 calories) per serve.

ABOVE: Easy Beef Curry. BELOW: Meatloaf with Basil Sauce. OPPOSITE PAGE: Top: Cheese-Topped Lasagne; bottom: Cannelloni with Tasty Mince Filling

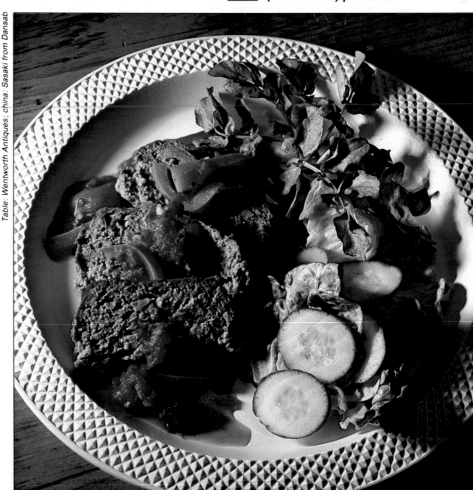

CHEESE-TOPPED LASAGNE

Meat sauce can be made a day ahead then covered and refrigerated, or it can be frozen for 3 months. Lasagne can be made a day ahead to the stage of cooking, then covered and refrigerated but it is not suitable to freeze at this stage. This recipe is not suitable to microwave.

100g lasagne noodles
¾ cup ricotta cheese (150g)
1 tablespoon grated parmesan cheese
1 egg white
1 tablespoon chopped fresh parsley
MEAT SAUCE
1 small onion (80g), finely chopped
1 clove garlic, crushed
1 tablespoon water
150g lean minced beef
425g can tomatoes
1 tablespoon tomato paste
¼ teaspoon dried basil leaves
¼ teaspoon dried oregano leaves
¼ teaspoon sugar

Prepare lasagne as directed on packet. Arrange single layer of lasagne over base of 15cm x 25cm ovenproof dish, top with meat sauce, then another layer of lasagne. Process cheeses, egg white and parsley until smooth, spread mixture evenly over lasagne. Bake in moderate oven for about 20 minutes.
Meat Sauce: Combine onion, garlic and water in saucepan, stir over heat until onion is soft, add mince, stir over heat until mince is well browned, stir in undrained, crushed tomatoes and remaining ingredients. Bring to the boil, reduce heat, simmer, uncovered, for about 20 minutes or until sauce is slightly thickened.
Serves 4.

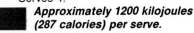
Approximately 1155 kilojoules (275 calories) per serve.

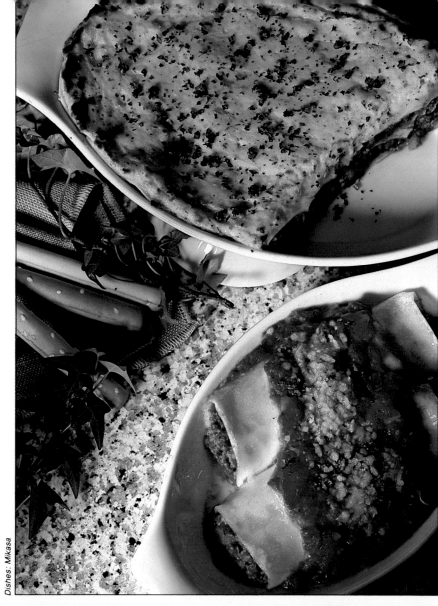

Dishes: Mikasa

CANNELLONI WITH TASTY MINCE FILLING

This recipe is not suitable to freeze.

¼ teaspoon oil
8 cannelloni shells
1 tablespoon grated parmesan cheese
TASTY MINCE FILLING
1 teaspoon oil
1 clove garlic, crushed
1 small onion (80g), finely chopped
300g lean minced beef
¼ teaspoon dried oregano leaves
1 medium tomato (100g), peeled, chopped
2 tablespoons tomato paste
TOMATO SAUCE
2 tablespoons water
1 small onion (80g), finely chopped
425g can tomatoes
pinch dried oregano leaves
2 teaspoons chopped fresh parsley

Drop cannelloni gradually into a large saucepan of boiling water, add oil and cook until cannelloni are tender, drain, place into bowl of warm water. Fill drained cannelloni with filling. Place in single layer in ovenproof dish, top with sauce, sprinkle with cheese and bake in moderate oven for about 30 minutes (or microwave on HIGH for about 10 minutes).
Tasty Mince Filling: Heat oil in frying pan, add garlic and onion, stir constantly over heat until onion is soft (or microwave on HIGH for about 3 minutes). Add mince, cook, stirring, until browned (or microwave on HIGH for about 2 minutes). Add oregano, tomato and tomato paste, cook, uncovered, for 5 minutes (or microwave on HIGH for about 2 minutes).
Tomato Sauce: Heat water in small saucepan, add onion, cook until soft, add undrained, crushed tomatoes and oregano. Bring to the boil, reduce heat, simmer, uncovered, for about 5 minutes or until slightly thickened, add parsley, mix well.
Serves 4.

Approximately 1200 kilojoules (287 calories) per serve.

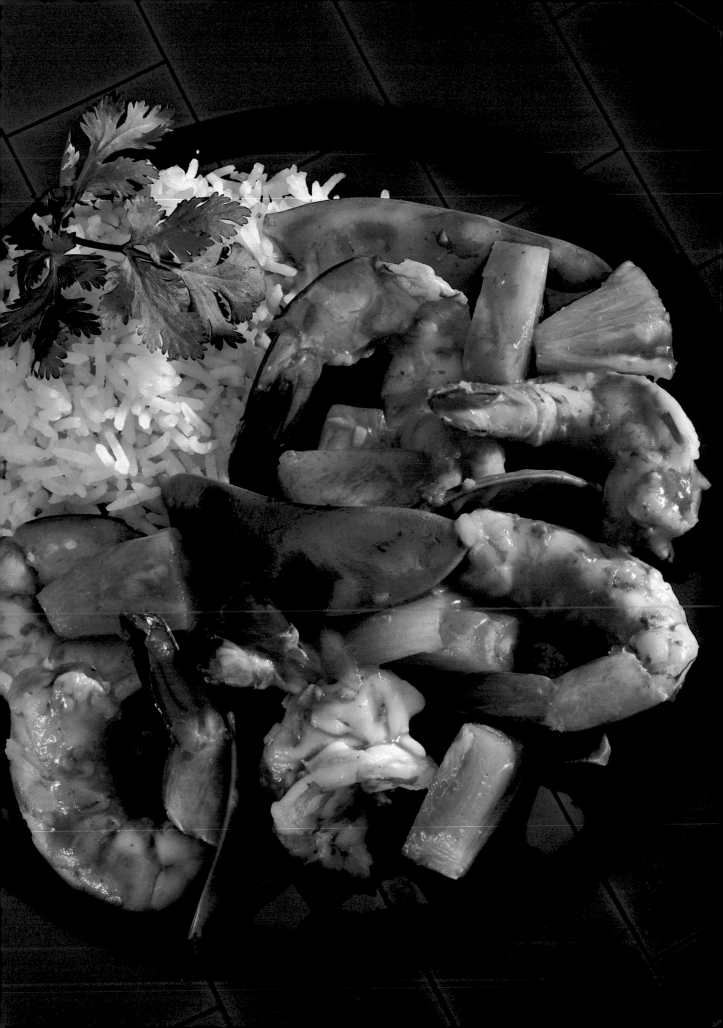

SEAFOOD

Seafood has wonderful nutritive value, is simple to prepare and cook, but, best of all, it is low in kilojoules. Fish fillets should be free from skin and bones before cooking; however, fish cutlets or steaks often have a central bone and skin intact which hold the piece of fish together during cooking. Check individual recipes for instructions on how to prepare the fish. Shellfish are low in kilojoules but prawns are sometimes restricted in low-cholesterol diets; if in doubt, check with your doctor or nutritionist.

SWEET AND SOUR PRAWNS

You will need to cook two-thirds cup of rice for this recipe. This dish is not suitable to freeze.

750g cooked king prawns
⅓ cup water
1 medium onion (120g), coarsely chopped
2 cloves garlic, crushed
1 teaspoon grated fresh ginger
3 teaspoons cornflour
½ cup water, extra
¼ cup tomato sauce
¼ cup brown vinegar
1 tablespoon sugar
200g snow peas
440g can unsweetened pineapple pieces, drained
2 cups cooked rice

Remove heads and shells and devein prawns, leaving tails intact. Heat water in a frying pan, add onion, garlic and ginger, stir constantly over heat until onion is soft (or microwave on HIGH about 5 minutes).

Blend cornflour with extra water, add tomato sauce, vinegar and sugar; stir into onion mixture. Stir constantly over heat until mixture boils and thickens (or microwave on HIGH for about 3 minutes).

Add snow peas, reduce heat, simmer, uncovered, for 3 minutes (or microwave on HIGH about 2 minutes), add prawns and pineapple, heat through. Serve with rice.
Serves 4.

Approximately 1150 kilojoules (274 calories) per serve.

ORANGE TERIYAKI FISH

We used perch fillets. This recipe is not suitable to freeze or microwave.

4 x 125g white fish fillets
1 teaspoon grated orange rind
½ cup orange juice
2 green shallots, chopped
1 tablespoon teriyaki sauce
1 teaspoon grated fresh ginger
1 teaspoon cornflour
1 tablespoon water

Combine fish, orange rind and juice, shallots, teriyaki sauce and ginger in a large bowl; cover, refrigerate 1 hour. Place fish mixture into a large frying pan, bring to the boil, reduce heat, simmer covered, for a few minutes or until fish is tender. Lift fish from orange mixture, place fish onto serving plate, keep warm.

Stir blended cornflour and water into orange mixture, stir constantly until sauce boils and thickens. Pour over fish before serving.
Serves 4.

Approximately 530 kilojoules (127 calories) per serve.

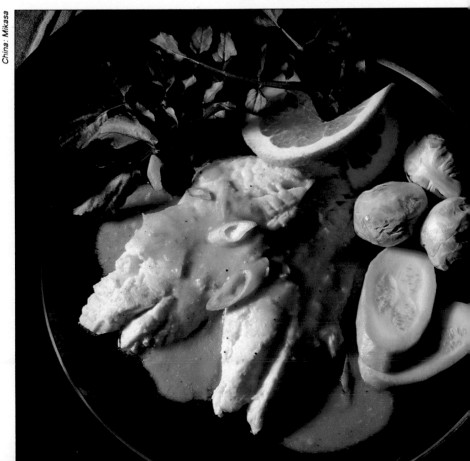

China: Mikasa

Plate: Sasaki from Dansab

LEFT: Sweet and Sour Prawns. RIGHT: Orange Teriyaki Fish

LETTUCE FISH PARCELS

We used bream fillets for this recipe. The dish can be frozen for 1 month.

4 white fish fillets (500g)
4 lettuce leaves
1 cup skim milk
½ cup dry white wine
2 tablespoons cornflour
½ cup water
2 teaspoons French mustard
1 small chicken stock cube,
**   crumbled**
2 tablespoons chopped fresh parsley
2 tablespoons grated parmesan
**   cheese**
½ cup stale wholemeal breadcrumbs
2 tablespoons grated parmesan
**   cheese, extra**
1 tablespoon chopped fresh parsley,
**   extra**
1 teaspoon paprika

Place fish in frying pan of cold water, bring to the boil, reduce heat, cover, simmer for 5 minutes (or microwave on HIGH for about 3 minutes). Drop lettuce leaves into a saucepan of boiling water, drain immediately, place into a bowl of iced water, drain. Wrap each fish fillet in a lettuce leaf.

Combine milk and wine in a saucepan, stir in blended cornflour and water. Stir constantly over heat until sauce boils and thickens. Add mustard, stock cube, parsley and cheese, stir lightly.

Place fish rolls in an ovenproof dish, top with sauce. Mix breadcrumbs, extra cheese, extra parsley and paprika together in bowl, sprinkle over sauce. Bake in moderate oven for about 15 minutes or until lightly browned (or microwave on HIGH about 5 minutes).
Serves 4.

Approximately 920 kilojoules (220 calories) per serve.

FISH AND SPINACH ROLLS

We used bream fillets for this dish. This recipe is not suitable to freeze.

4 large spinach (silver beet) leaves
**   (100g)**
4 x 125g white fish fillets
180g ricotta cheese
1 tablespoon grated parmesan
**   cheese**
1 teaspoon butter
SAUCE
1 teaspoon butter
1 clove garlic, crushed
1 small onion (80g), chopped
2 medium ripe tomatoes (200g),
**   peeled, chopped**
1 small chicken stock cube, crumbled
½ cup water
2 tablespoons dry white wine
¼ teaspoon dried oregano leaves

Remove white stalks from spinach. Cut each leaf in half lengthwise, drop leaves into a saucepan of boiling water, drain immediately, place into a bowl of iced water; lift leaves out and drain.

Place fish, skin side down on bench. Spread each fillet evenly with combined cheeses. Place each piece of fish between 2 pieces of spinach, roll up firmly, secure with toothpicks.

Place rolls in ovenproof dish, dot with butter, cover, bake in moderate oven 20 minutes (or microwave on HIGH for about 5 minutes) until just tender. Cool 1 minute before slicing; serve with sauce.

Sauce: Heat butter in small frying pan, add garlic and onion, stir constantly over heat until onion is soft. Add tomatoes, stock cube, water and wine.

Table: Freedom Furniture; china: Pillivuyt from Accoutrement

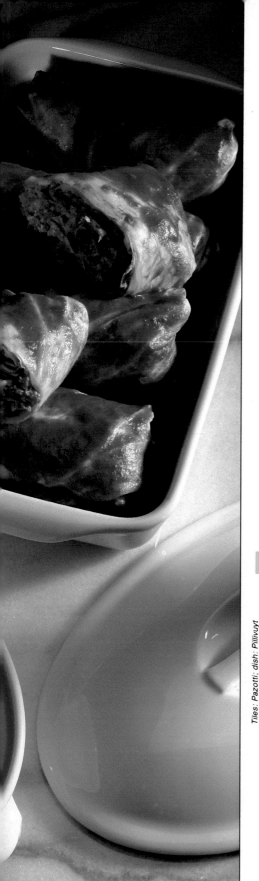

SALMON AND FETTA CHEESE CABBAGE ROLLS

This recipe is not suitable to freeze. The salmon can be substituted with tuna, if preferred.

8 cabbage leaves
440g can salmon, drained
60g fetta cheese
4 green shallots, chopped
1 medium carrot (120g), finely grated
1 medium stick celery (80g), sliced
1 tablespoon lemon juice
TOMATO SAUCE
3 teaspoons cornflour
1½ cups canned tomato juice
2 teaspoons Worcestershire sauce
1 teaspoon light soya sauce

Boil, steam or microwave cabbage leaves until just tender, drain, cut away thick parts from base of leaves.

Remove skin and bones from salmon, flake salmon with fork. Stir in crumbled cheese, shallots, carrot, celery and lemon juice. Place an equal portion of salmon mixture on each cabbage leaf, roll leaves firmly, tucking in edges.

Place rolls in single layer in ovenproof dish, top with tomato sauce, cover, bake in moderate oven for about 45 minutes (or microwave on HIGH for about 15 minutes). Serve with tomato sauce.

Tomato Sauce: Blend cornflour with combined tomato juice and sauces in a saucepan, stir constantly over heat until sauce boils and thickens.

Serves 4.

Approximately 1200 kilojoules (287 calories) per serve.
If using tuna, 995 kilojoules (237 calories) per serve.

OCTOPUSES IN RED WINE

Casserole can be frozen for up to 2 months; it is not suitable to microwave.

750g baby octopuses
1 cup dry red wine
2 teaspoons oil
1 clove garlic, crushed
1 medium onion (120g), finely chopped
2 bacon rashers (80g), chopped
1 tablespoon pine nuts
425g can tomatoes
1 tablespoon lemon juice
1 tablespoon chopped fresh parsley

Prepare octopuses by cutting off the heads, just below the eyes. Remove beaks, rinse octopuses under cold water. Place octopuses and wine in a bowl, cover, refrigerate, marinate 4 hours or overnight.

Next day, drain octopuses, reserve 2 tablespoons of the wine marinade. Heat oil in a frying pan, add garlic, onion and bacon, stir constantly over heat until onion is soft. Add pine nuts, stir over heat a further 2 minutes. Add undrained, crushed tomatoes, lemon juice and reserved wine; bring to the boil, reduce heat, simmer, uncovered, 5 minutes.

Place octopuses in ovenproof dish, add tomato mixture, cover, bake in moderate oven for 1½ hours. Stir in parsley just before serving.

Serves 4.

Approximately 1080 kilojoules (258 calories) per serve.

LEFT: Clockwise from top left: Fish and Spinach Rolls; Salmon and Fetta Cheese Cabbage Rolls; Lettuce Fish Parcels.
BELOW: Octopuses in Red Wine

Tiles: Pazotti; dish: Pillivuyt

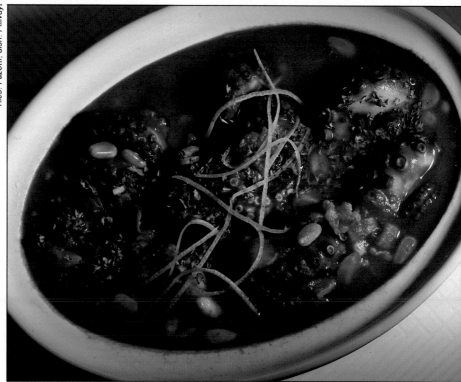

Bring to the boil, reduce heat and simmer, uncovered, for about 5 minutes, or until mixture thickens slightly. Blend or process tomato mixture until smooth; stir in oregano.

Serves 4.

Approximately 865 kilojoules (207 calories) per serve.

CURRIED FISH WITH GARLIC VEGETABLES

We used bream fillets for this recipe. This dish is not suitable to freeze.

400g white fish fillets
1 tablespoon plain flour
2 teaspoons curry powder
2 teaspoons oil
1 tablespoon lemon juice
1 small onion (80g), finely chopped
1 clove garlic, crushed
1 cup water
2 green shallots, chopped
2 medium zucchini (300g), sliced
1 medium stick celery (80g), sliced

Cut fish into strips, toss in combined flour and curry powder. Heat oil in frying pan, add lemon juice and fish and cook until lightly browned on all sides (or microwave on HIGH for about 2 minutes). Remove fish from pan.

Add onion, garlic, water, shallots, zucchini and celery to pan, cook, stirring, until vegetables are just tender (or microwave on HIGH, using half the water, for about 5 minutes). Serve the vegetables over fish.

Serves 4.

Approximately 560 kilojoules (133 calories) per serve.

SAUCY CURRIED FISH

We used bream fillets for this recipe. The fish rolls and sauce can be prepared for baking up to 3 hours ahead. This recipe is not suitable to freeze.

2 bacon rashers (80g)
125g mushrooms, finely chopped
2 green shallots, finely chopped
2 teaspoons French mustard
8 x 90g white fish fillets
SAUCE
2 teaspoons butter
1 teaspoon curry powder
1 medium onion (120g), finely chopped
2 tablespoons sultanas
1 small chicken stock cube, crumbled
2 teaspoons cornflour
1 cup water

Grill or microwave bacon until crisp; chop bacon finely. Combine bacon in bowl with mushrooms, shallots and mustard; mix well. Divide bacon mixture evenly over fish fillets, roll up firmly, secure with toothpicks.

Place rolls in ovenproof dish, cover, bake in moderate oven for about 30 minutes, or until fish is tender (or microwave on HIGH for about 10 minutes). Remove the toothpicks and top rolls with curry sauce before serving.

Sauce: Melt butter in small saucepan, add curry powder and onion, cook until onion is soft (or microwave on HIGH for about 5 minutes), add sultanas and stock cube then blended cornflour and water, stir constantly over heat until sauce boils and thickens (or microwave on HIGH for about 3 minutes).

Serves 4.

Approximately 1160 kilojoules (277 calories) per serve.

FISH WITH ALMONDS IN TOMATO HERB SAUCE

We used bream fillets in this recipe. The sauce can be made up to two days before it is required. This recipe is not suitable to freeze.

¼ cup flaked almonds
8 x 125g white fish fillets
⅓ cup lemon juice
TOMATO HERB SAUCE
⅓ cup water
1 medium onion (120g), finely chopped
1 clove garlic, crushed
425g can tomatoes
¼ cup dry red wine
1 teaspoon dried basil leaves
¼ cup chopped fresh parsley

Toast almonds on oven tray in moderate oven for about 5 minutes.

Brush fish with lemon juice, grill on both sides until tender (or microwave on HIGH for about 6 minutes). Serve with sauce, sprinkle with almonds.

Tomato Herb Sauce: Place water in frying pan, add onion and garlic, stir constantly over heat until onion is soft (or microwave on HIGH about 5 minutes). Add undrained, crushed tomatoes, wine and basil, bring to the boil, reduce heat, simmer uncovered, for 5 minutes or until sauce is slightly thickened (or microwave on HIGH for about 5 minutes), stir in parsley.

Serves 4.

Approximately 1125 kilojoules (268 calories) per serve.

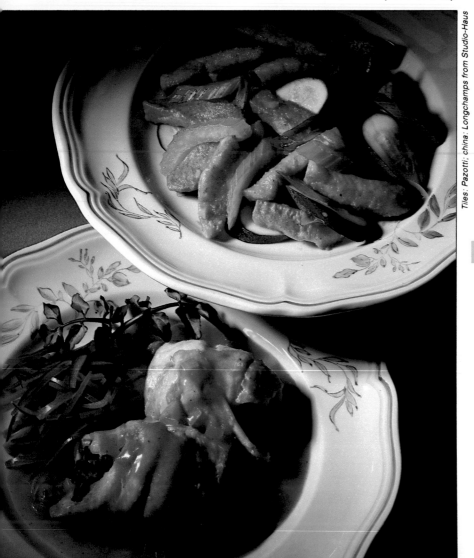

Tiles: Pazotti; china: Longchamps from Studio-Haus

LEFT: Top: Curried Fish with Garlic Vegetables; bottom: Saucy Curried Fish.
RIGHT: Top: Fish with Almonds in Tomato Herb Sauce; bottom: Stir-Fried Fish with Ginger

Tiles: Pazotti; china: Lifestyle Imports

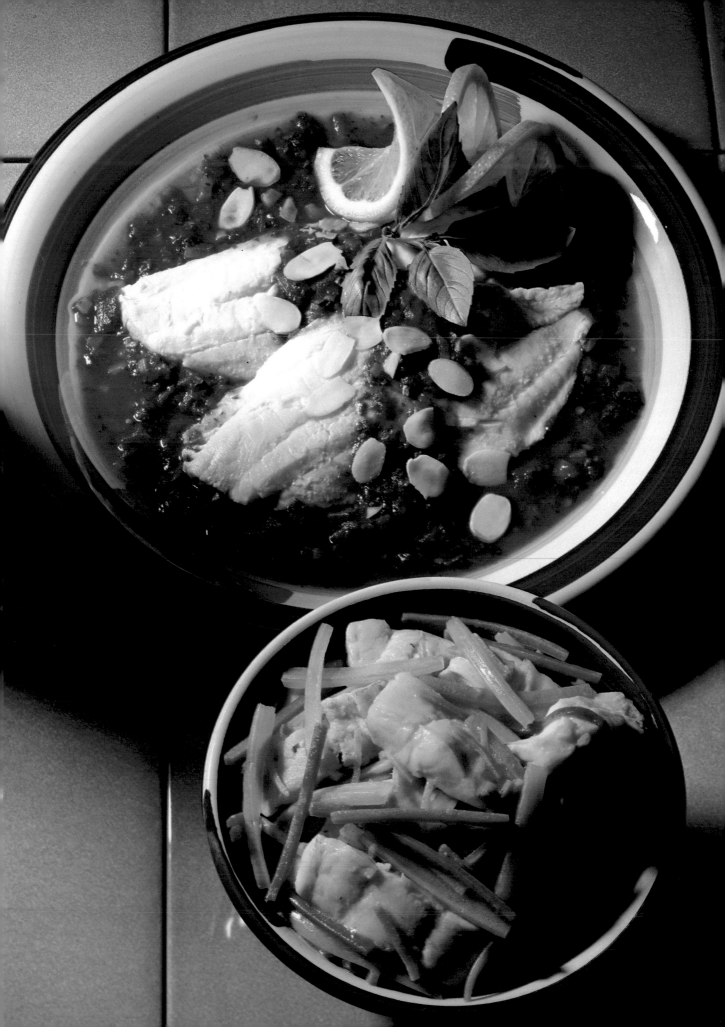

STIR-FRIED FISH WITH GINGER

We used ling fish for this recipe; it is not suitable to freeze or microwave.

750g white fish fillets
2 medium carrots (240g)
2 small sticks celery (120g)
1cm piece fresh ginger, peeled
1 teaspoon cornflour
1 small chicken stock cube, crumbled
½ cup water
2 teaspoons oil
1 tablespoon oil, extra

Cut fish into chunks, cut carrots and celery into narrow strips. Cut ginger into wafer-thin slices, then into fine shreds. Blend cornflour and stock cube in bowl with water.

Heat oil in frying pan or wok, add carrots and celery, stir-fry over high heat for a few minutes, remove from pan. Heat extra oil in pan, add fish and ginger, stir-fry over high heat until fish is tender. Add vegetables and cornflour mixture; stir constantly over heat until sauce boils and thickens.

Serves 4.

Approximately 1005 kilojoules (240 calories) per serve.

BELOW: Chilli Prawn Kebabs. RIGHT: Top: Lemony Fish Cutlets; bottom: Mustard and Honeyed Fish

MUSTARD AND HONEYED FISH

We used redfish fillets for this recipe. This dish is not suitable to freeze.

8 small fish fillets (500g)
2 tablespoons grated parmesan cheese
SAUCE
2 teaspoons oil
1 tablespoon lemon juice
2 teaspoons French mustard
1 teaspoon honey
3 teaspoons cornflour
¾ cup water

Place fish onto griller tray, sprinkle fish with half the cheese. Grill fish for 3 minutes, turn fish carefully, sprinkle with remaining cheese, grill further 3 minutes (or microwave on HIGH for about 3 minutes). Serve with sauce.

Sauce: Combine oil, lemon juice, mustard and honey in a small saucepan; stir in blended cornflour and water, stir constantly over heat until sauce boils and thickens. Reduce heat, simmer uncovered, 1 minute (or microwave on HIGH about 1 minute).

Serves 4.

Approximately 670 kilojoules (160 calories) per serve.

LEMONY FISH CUTLETS

We used gemfish cutlets in this recipe. This dish is not suitable to freeze or microwave.

4 x 250g white fish cutlets
15g butter
1 small red pepper (100g), chopped
4 green shallots, finely chopped
⅔ cup stale breadcrumbs
2 tablespoons chopped fresh parsley
1 teaspoon grated lemon rind
2 tablespoons low oil mayonnaise
2 teaspoons butter, melted, extra
1 tablespoon lemon juice

Remove large bone from each cutlet. Heat butter in frying pan, add pepper and shallots, stir constantly over heat until pepper is soft. Remove from heat, stir in breadcrumbs, parsley, lemon rind and mayonnaise. Fill bone cavity in each cutlet with breadcrumb mixture.

Brush cutlets with combined extra butter and lemon juice, cook under hot griller until fish is tender, brushing occasionally with lemon juice mixture.

Serves 4.

Approximately 1255 kilojoules (300 calories) per serve.

CHILLI PRAWN KEBABS

Soak bamboo skewers in water for at least an hour to prevent burning during cooking. You will need to cook two-thirds cup of rice to serve with this recipe. This recipe is not suitable to freeze or microwave.

24 uncooked king prawns (700g)
1 clove garlic, crushed
½ cup tomato purée
1 tablespoon white vinegar
2 teaspoons Worcestershire sauce
2 teaspoons light soya sauce
2 small fresh red chillies, finely chopped
3 teaspoons sugar
¼ teaspoon chilli powder
1 large red pepper (225g)
2 teaspoons cornflour
⅓ cup water
2 cups cooked rice

Remove heads and shells, and devein prawns, leaving tails intact. Combine garlic, tomato purée, vinegar, sauces, chillies, sugar and chilli powder in large bowl, add prawns, cover; refrigerate several hours or overnight.

Cut pepper into 2cm pieces. Thread pepper and prawns alternately onto skewers, place under hot griller, grill until prawns are cooked, brushing occasionally with chilli mixture.

Blend cornflour with water, combine with remaining chilli mixture in saucepan, stir constantly over heat until mixture boils and thickens. Serve kebabs with rice, top with chilli sauce.

Serves 4.

Approximately 860 kilojoules (205 calories) per serve.

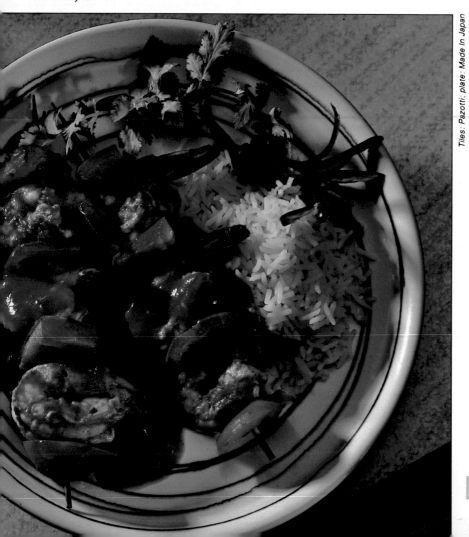

Tiles: Pazotti; plate: Made in Japan

Table: Freedom Furniture; china: Sasaki from Dansab

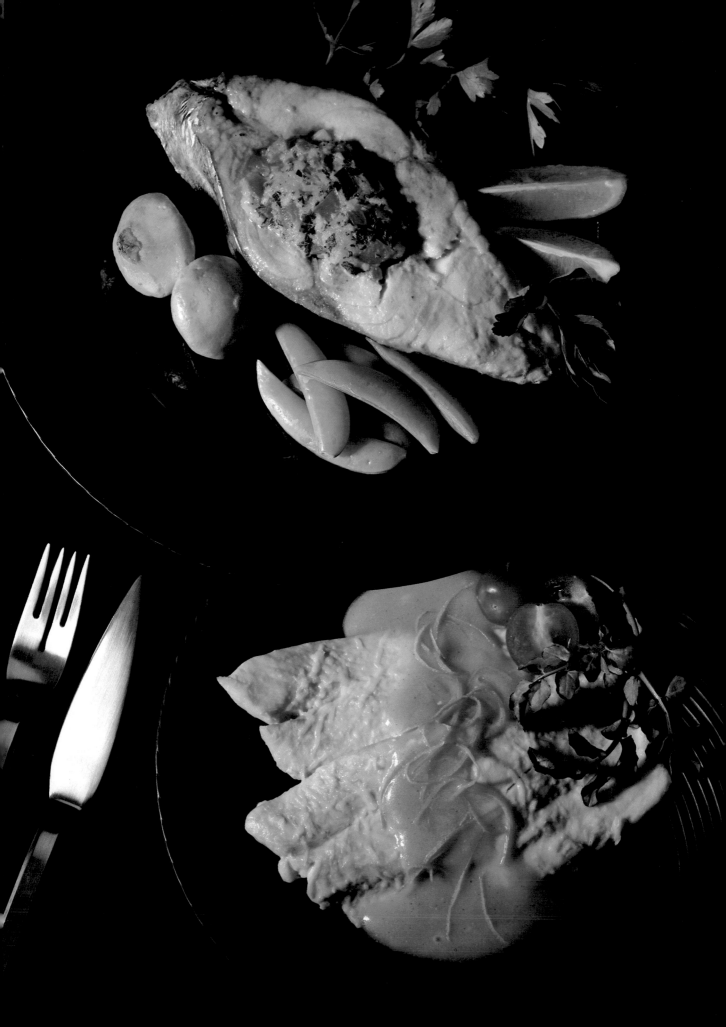

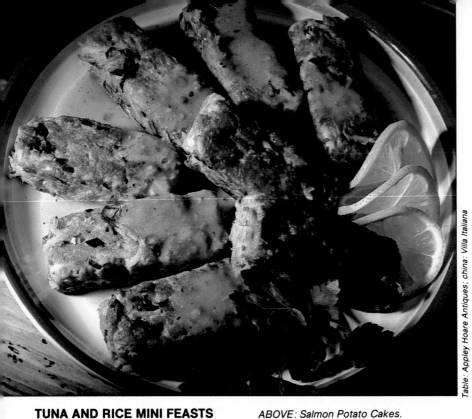

SALMON POTATO CAKES

Cakes are best made just before cooking, because potato will discolour on standing. This recipe is not suitable to freeze or microwave.

440g can salmon
2 medium potatoes (200g), coarsely grated
1 egg, lightly beaten
3 green shallots, sliced
2 teaspoons oil
SAUCE
1 teaspoon lemon juice
13g sachet low-joule vegetable soup mix

Drain salmon, reserve liquid, remove bones and skin from salmon.

Place salmon in bowl, mix in potatoes, egg and shallots. Divide mixture into 8 portions, pat into desired shape. Heat oil in a frying pan, add cakes, fry on each side until golden brown and firm. Serve with sauce.

Sauce: Combine reserved salmon liquid with enough water to measure half a cup liquid. Place in small saucepan with lemon juice, bring to the boil, stir in soup mix.

Serves 4.

Approximately 1080 kilojoules (258 calories) per serve.

Table: Appley Hoare Antiques; china: Villa Italiana

TUNA AND RICE MINI FEASTS

Peppers can be prepared to the stage of cooking, covered and refrigerated for up to 6 hours, if preferred. You will need to cook one-third cup of rice for this recipe; it is not suitable to freeze.

2 large green peppers (450g)
1 medium onion (120g), finely chopped
1 clove garlic, crushed
2 teaspoons water
425g can tomatoes
1 tablespoon tomato paste
¼ teaspoon dried basil leaves
¼ teaspoon dried oregano leaves
2 teaspoons chopped fresh parsley
185g can tuna in brine, drained
1 cup cooked brown rice
⅔ cup grated mozzarella cheese (60g)
2 teaspoons grated parmesan cheese

Cut peppers in half lengthways, remove and discard pith and seeds. Combine onion, garlic and water in saucepan, stir constantly over heat until onion is soft. Stir in undrained, crushed tomatoes, tomato paste and herbs, bring to the boil, reduce heat, simmer, uncovered, for about 10 minutes or until mixture is quite thick.

Remove from heat, stir in flaked tuna and rice.

Divide mixture evenly into pepper halves, place pepper halves onto oven tray, bake in moderate oven for about 15 minutes (or microwave on HIGH for about 4 minutes). Sprinkle pepper halves with combined cheeses, bake further 10 minutes (or microwave on HIGH for about 2 minutes).

Serves 4.

Approximately 765 kilojoules (183 calories) per serve.

ABOVE: Salmon Potato Cakes.
OPPOSITE PAGE: Top: Sweet and Sour Fish; bottom: Stir-Fried Ginger Seafood.
BELOW: Tuna and Rice Mini Feasts

Dish: John Dermer, Pottery, Yackandandah, Vic.

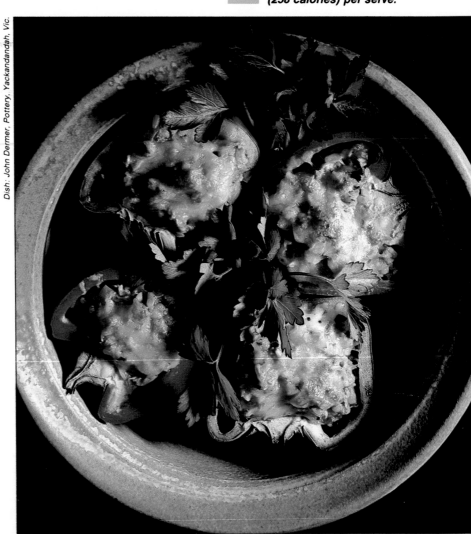

MUSSELS WITH LEEK AND TOMATO SAUCE

This recipe is not suitable to freeze or microwave.

24 mussels (1kg)
1 tablespoon oil
1 clove garlic, crushed
1 large leek (250g), thinly sliced
425g can tomatoes
½ cup dry white wine
½ teaspoon dried oregano leaves
½ teaspoon sugar
1 tablespoon chopped fresh parsley
5 pitted black olives, chopped

Scrub mussels under cold water, remove beards. Heat oil in a large frying pan, add garlic and leek, cook gently for about 15 minutes, or until leek is soft. Add undrained, crushed tomatoes, wine, oregano and sugar, bring to the boil, add mussels, cover, boil 2 minutes. Remove mussels as they open and place in serving bowls; discard any mussels that do not open.

Boil sauce, uncovered, for about 5 minutes or until thickened, stir in parsley and olives. Pour sauce over mussels before serving.

Serves 4.

Approximately 490 kilojoules (117 calories) per serve.

TOP RIGHT: Mussels with Leek and Tomato Sauce. BOTTOM RIGHT: Stir-Fried Pimiento Prawns

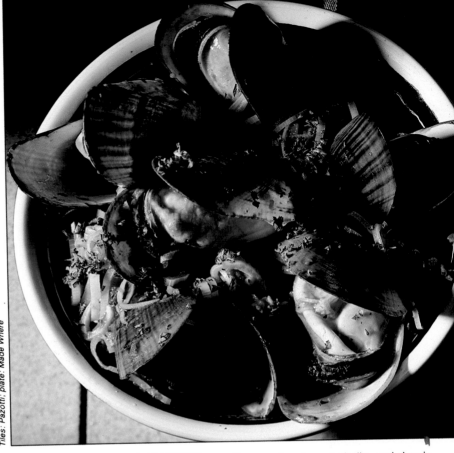

Tiles: Pazotti; plate: Made Where

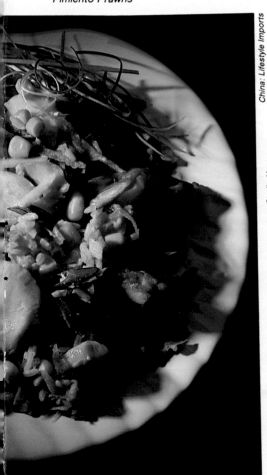

China: Lifestyle Imports

STIR-FRIED PIMIENTO PRAWNS

This recipe is not suitable to freeze or microwave.

40 medium uncooked prawns (1¼kg)
2 teaspoons oil
2 tablespoons dry white wine
½ cup canned beef consommé
1 tablespoon teriyaki sauce
1 drained canned pimiento (60g), finely chopped
1 teaspoon grated fresh ginger
4 green shallots, sliced
1 tablespoon canned tomato purée
3 teaspoons cornflour
1 tablespoon water

Remove heads and shells, and devein prawns, leaving tails intact. Heat oil in wok or frying pan, add prawns, stir-fry over high heat until prawns are almost cooked. Stir in wine and consommé, then teriyaki sauce, pimiento, ginger, shallots and tomato purée, simmer 2 minutes. Stir in blended cornflour and water; stir constantly until sauce boils and thickens.

Serves 4.

Approximately 840 kilojoules (200 calories) per serve.

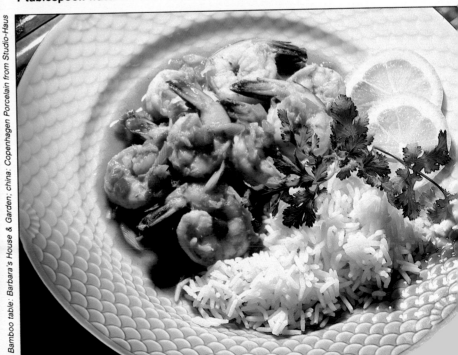

Bamboo table: Barbara's House & Garden; china: Copenhagen Porcelain from Studio-Haus.

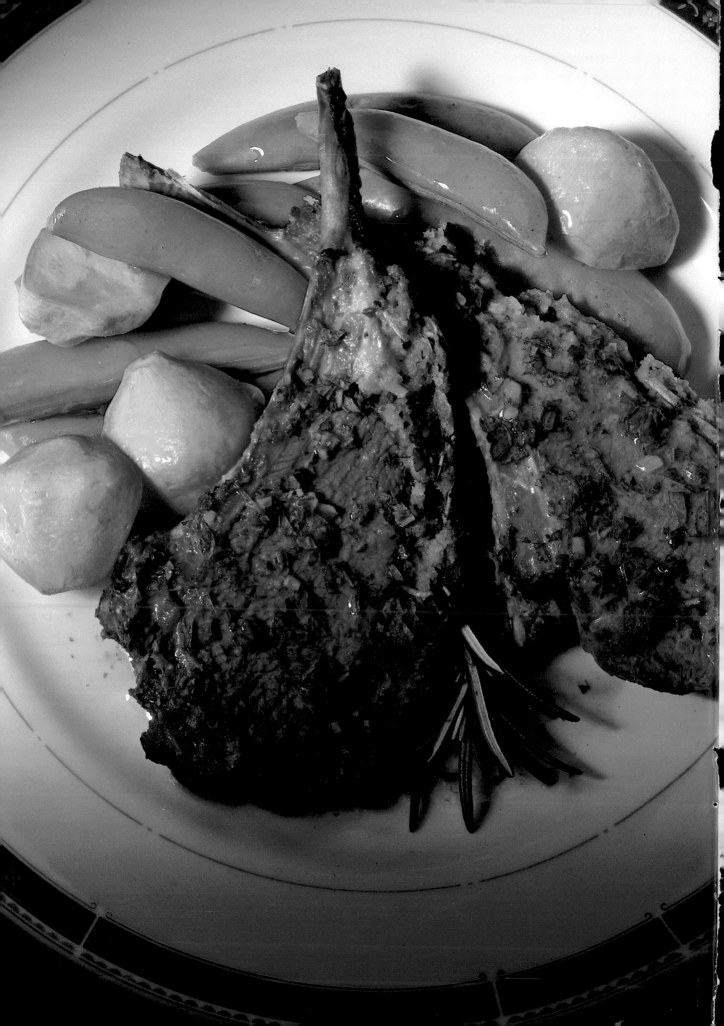

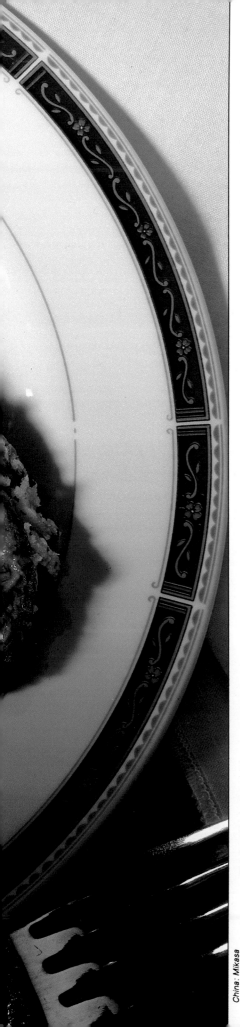

MAIN COURSES
LAMB

Lamb is full of flavour and can be a wonderful food if you are watching your weight. Buy lean lamb and trim away as much fat as possible before cooking.

MINTED LEMON LAMB

This recipe is not suitable to freeze or microwave.

1 cup stale breadcrumbs
1 teaspoon grated lemon rind
2 teaspoons chopped fresh mint
1 teaspoon dried rosemary leaves
½ teaspoon sugar
1 teaspoon oil
2 tablespoons lemon juice,
**   approximately**
4 racks of lamb (2 cutlets each)
**   (600g)**
LEMON MINT SAUCE
2 teaspoons butter
1 teaspoon grated lemon rind
¼ cup lemon juice
1 tablespoon chopped fresh mint

Combine breadcrumbs, lemon rind, mint, rosemary, sugar and oil in bowl, add enough lemon juice to bind ingredients together. Pat mixture firmly along back of cutlets. Place cutlets (crumb side up) on rack over baking dish, bake in moderate oven for about 30 minutes. Serve with sauce.

Lemon Mint Sauce: Combine all ingredients in saucepan, stir constantly over heat until mixture boils.

Serves 4.

 Approximately 1195 kilojoules (285 calories) per serve.

LEFT: Minted Lemon Lamb. BELOW: Springtime Lamb Casserole

SPRINGTIME LAMB CASSEROLE

Casserole can be cooked a day ahead or frozen for up to 2 months.

4 lamb chump chops (600g)
1 tablespoon paprika
35g packet spring vegetable soup
1 cup dry white wine
2 cups water
1 clove garlic, crushed
2 tablespoons chopped fresh parsley
2 medium potatoes (200g), chopped
2 large carrots (400g), sliced
3 medium sticks celery (240g),
**   chopped**
2 small green peppers (200g),
**   chopped**
2 small red peppers (200g), chopped
1½ tablespoons cornflour
¼ cup water, extra

Remove bones from chops, cut meat into cubes, mix well with paprika. Combine dry soup with wine, water, garlic and parsley in ovenproof dish, add lamb, potatoes, carrots, celery and peppers. Bake in moderate oven for about 1 hour (or microwave on HIGH for about 20 minutes) or until tender.

Blend cornflour with extra water, add to lamb mixture, return to oven for about 15 minutes (or microwave on HIGH for about 5 minutes) or until mixture boils and thickens.

Serves 4.

Approximately 1245 kilojoules (297 calories) per serve.

Dish & napkin: Accoutrement

China: Mikasa

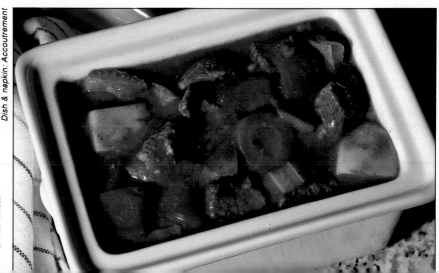

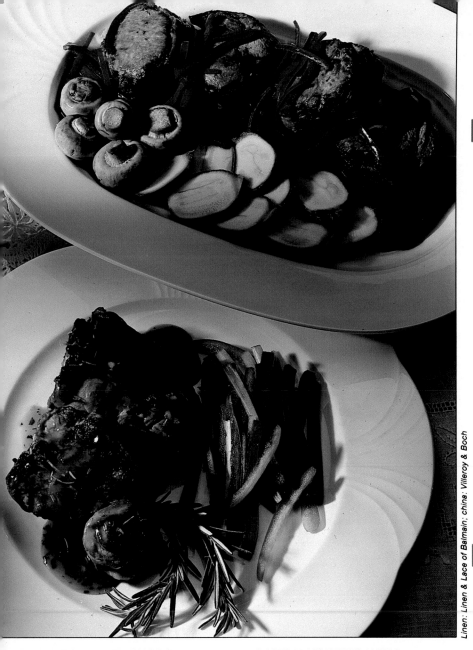

heat until sauce boils and thickens, add pepper, simmer 1 minute. Remove string from noisettes before serving with sauce.

Serves 4.

Approximately 1190 kilojoules (284 calories) per serve.

HEARTY LAMB CASSEROLE

This casserole can be frozen for 2 months; it is unsuitable to microwave.

4 x 300g lamb shanks
1 medium onion (120g), sliced
2 small sticks celery (120g), sliced
2 medium carrots (240g), sliced
1 cup water
1 cup tomato juice
½ cup dry white wine
1 clove garlic, crushed
1 small chicken stock cube, crumbled
1 teaspoon paprika
1 teaspoon ground ginger

Heat a non-stick frying pan, add shanks, cook until well browned all over. Place shanks, onion, celery and carrots in a large ovenproof dish. Add water, tomato juice, wine, garlic, stock cube, paprika and ginger, cover, bake in moderate oven for about 2½ hours or until lamb is tender. Cool casserole, refrigerate overnight.

Next day lift off fat, reheat casserole on top of stove, or in moderate oven for about 30 minutes.

Serves 4.

Approximately 1250 kilojoules (298 calories) per serve.

Linen: Linen & Lace of Balmain; china: Villeroy & Boch

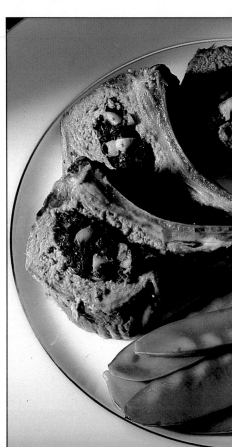

HERBED LAMB CHOPS

This recipe is not suitable to freeze or microwave.

1 clove garlic, crushed
4 x 100g lamb loin chops
1 teaspoon cornflour
½ cup water
1 tablespoon chopped fresh mint
1 teaspoon dried rosemary leaves
2 teaspoons brown vinegar
½ teaspoon sugar
1 tablespoon mint jelly

Heat a non-stick frying pan, add garlic and chops, cook until chops are well browned and cooked as desired, remove chops from pan, keep warm.

Combine blended cornflour and water in bowl with remaining ingredients, add to pan, stir constantly over heat until mixture boils and thickens. Return chops to pan, heat until chops are glazed all over.

Serves 4.

Approximately 1255 kilojoules (300 calories) per serve.

LAMB NOISETTES WITH RED WINE SAUCE

Noisette, French for hazelnut, is the name given to a small piece of lamb or mutton, such as a chop, with bone removed and meat fastened into a round shape. This dish can be prepared several hours before cooking, but is not suitable to freeze or microwave.

4 x 100g lamb loin chops
½ teaspoon dried oregano leaves
1 small beef stock cube, crumbled
½ cup water
½ cup dry red wine
1 teaspoon cornflour
¼ cup water, extra
½ medium red pepper (75g), sliced

Cut bones from chops, sprinkle inside of chop tail with oregano, wrap tail around chop, secure with string. Grill chops until cooked as desired. Combine stock cube, water and wine in a saucepan, bring to the boil; reduce heat, simmer, uncovered, until reduced by half. Blend cornflour with extra water, add to pan, stir constantly over

SPINACH-SEASONED LAMB

Lamb can be seasoned several hours in advance, then cooked just before serving. Cover exposed bones of cutlets with foil to prevent bones from burning. This recipe is not suitable to microwave.

2 racks of lamb (6 cutlets on each) (900g)
SEASONING
5 spinach (silver beet) leaves (100g)
1 small onion (80g), chopped
1 tablespoon currants
1 tablespoon tomato paste
1 clove garlic, crushed
¼ teaspoon ground cinnamon

Cut a pocket in each rack along the edge where meat is closest to the bone; leave 1½cm at each end uncut. Spoon seasoning into each pocket, secure opening with toothpicks. Bake in hot oven for about 20 minutes, lower temperature to moderate and bake further 10 to 20 minutes, depending on how you prefer lamb cooked. Remove toothpicks from lamb, cut into cutlets, allowing 3 cutlets per person.

Seasoning: Remove centre stalks from spinach leaves. Place onion in a saucepan of boiling water, boil 5 minutes, add spinach, drain immediately, press out as much liquid as possible, chop spinach and onion finely. Combine spinach mixture in bowl with currants, tomato paste, garlic and cinnamon and mix well.

Serves 4.

■ Approximately 1180 kilojoules (282 calories) per serve.

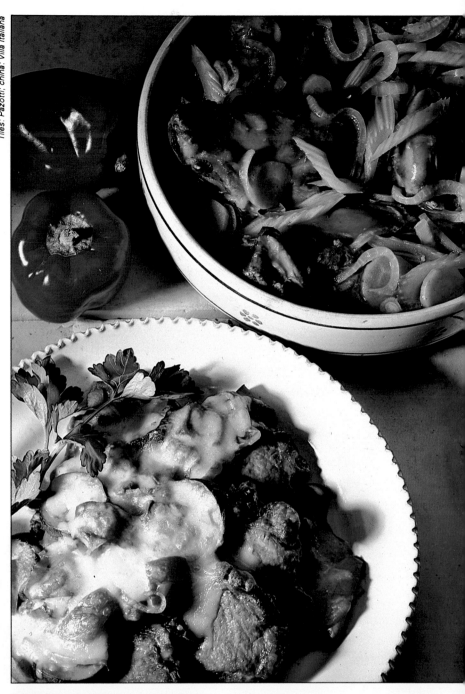

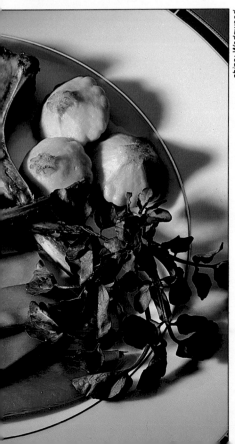

CHEESE-TOPPED RATATOUILLE LAMB CUTLETS

Ratatouille, a vegetable dish that originated in Provence, can be made a day ahead. This recipe is not suitable to freeze or microwave.

1 small eggplant (250g)
salt
1 small onion (80g), thinly sliced
2 small zucchini (200g), chopped
1 small red pepper (100g), chopped
1 clove garlic, crushed
2 tablespoons water
1 small chicken stock cube, crumbled
½ cup tomato purée
¼ teaspoon dried basil leaves
¼ teaspoon dried oregano leaves
4 x 100g lamb cutlets
60g mozzarella cheese, thinly sliced

Cut eggplant into 1cm cubes, sprinkle with salt, stand 20 minutes, rinse well under cold water, drain.

Combine eggplant, onion, zucchini, pepper, garlic and water in saucepan, stir constantly over heat until onion is soft. Stir in stock cube, tomato purée and herbs, bring to the boil, reduce heat, simmer, uncovered, 10 minutes, stirring occasionally.

Grill cutlets until browned and tender. Top cutlets with vegetable mixture and cheese, grill until cheese melts.

Serves 4.

■ Approximately 820 kilojoules (195 calories) per serve.

FAR LEFT: Top: Lamb Noisettes with Red Wine Sauce; bottom: Herbed Lamb Chops. LEFT: Spinach-Seasoned Lamb. ABOVE: Top: Hearty Lamb Casserole; bottom: Cheese-Topped Ratatouille Lamb Cutlets

Tiles: Pazotti; china: Villa Italiana

china: Wedgwood

VEGETARIAN

Vegetables lend themselves perfectly to satisfying, low-kilojoule main courses with their varieties of flavours and colours. Our recipes are planned carefully for well-balanced nutrition. You will find more ideas for complete, vegetable-based meals in the sections for Entrees and Side Dishes in this book.

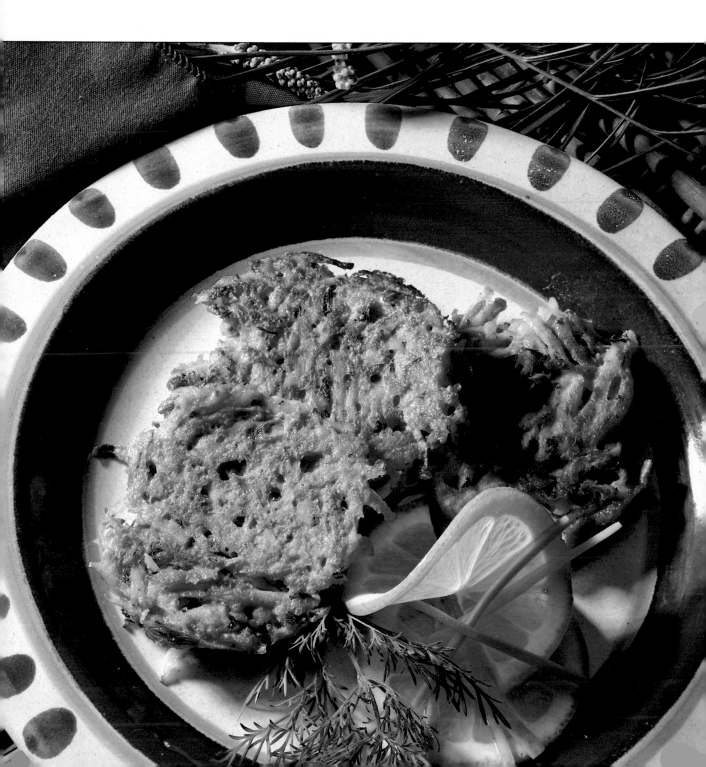

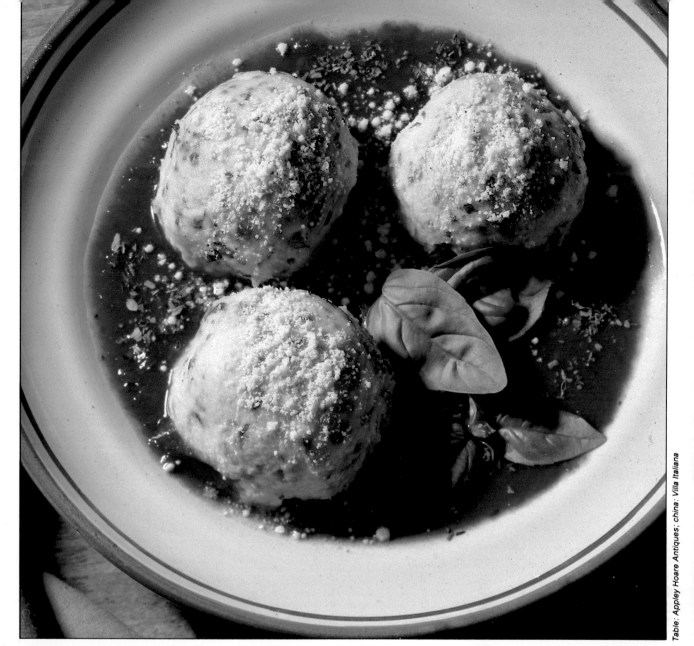

CRISPY CARROT AND POTATO PANCAKES

This recipe is not suitable to freeze or microwave.

2 large potatoes (370g), finely grated
2 large carrots (400g), finely grated
6 green shallots, chopped
2 tablespoons chopped fresh parsley
⅓ cup skim milk
2 eggs, lightly beaten
2 tablespoons wholemeal plain flour
1 teaspoon ground cumin

Rinse grated potato under cold water, squeeze out as much excess liquid as possible. Combine potatoes, carrots, shallots, parsley, milk, eggs, flour and cumin in a bowl, mix well. Drop 2 tablespoons of mixture into a lightly greased frying pan, cook over heat for about 5 minutes on each side, or until golden brown and vegetables are tender. Repeat with remaining mixture, making 12 pancakes.

Serves 4.

Approximately 685 kilojoules (164 calories) per serve.

SPINACH AND RICOTTA GNOCCHI

The traditional base of potatoes and flour is varied here with spinach and ricotta cheese. Gnocchi are not suitable to freeze or microwave.

12 spinach (silver beet) leaves (240g)
1¼ cups ricotta cheese (250g)
⅓ cup grated parmesan cheese (30g)
1 egg, lightly beaten
¼ teaspoon ground nutmeg
1½ tablespoons plain flour
1 teaspoon grated parmesan cheese, extra
TOMATO SAUCE
425g can tomatoes
2 teaspoons sugar
1 teaspoon dried oregano leaves

Remove stalks from spinach. Boil, steam or microwave leaves until tender, drain, squeeze out excess liquid, chop finely.

Combine spinach in bowl with ricotta, parmesan, egg and nutmeg, mix well. Roll into 12 balls, dust with flour. Bring a large saucepan of water to the boil. Using a spoon, place balls gently into the water, reduce heat slightly, simmer for about 2 minutes, or until balls rise to the surface of the water. Remove gnocchi with a slotted spoon, drain, serve immediately with sauce. Sprinkle with extra cheese.

Tomato Sauce: Blend or process undrained tomatoes until smooth, strain, heat in a saucepan with sugar and oregano (or microwave on HIGH for about 3 minutes).

Serves 4.

Approximately 835 kilojoules (200 calories) per serve.

ABOVE: Spinach and Ricotta Gnocchi.
LEFT: Crispy Carrot and Potato Pancakes

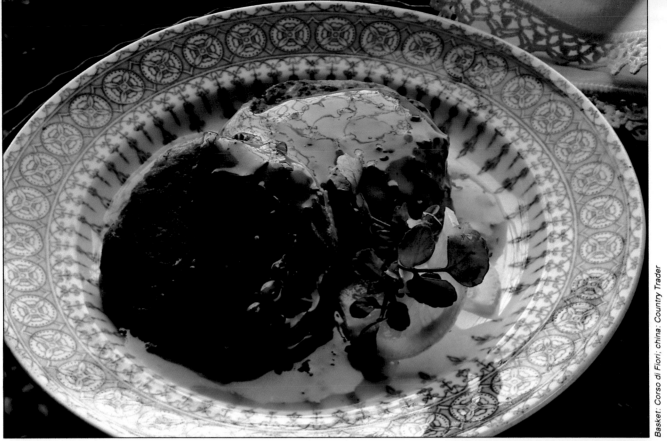

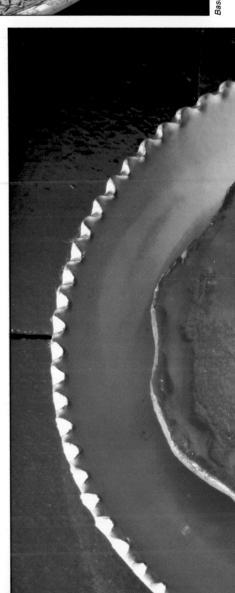

SWEET POTATO CAKES WITH FRESH HERB SAUCE

This recipe is not suitable to freeze or microwave.

2 small kumara (orange sweet potato) (300g), chopped
3 small potatoes (225g)
2 green shallots, chopped
1 egg, beaten
1 tablespoon oil
FRESH HERB SAUCE
1 cup water
1 small chicken stock cube, crumbled
1 tablespoon chopped fresh parsley
1 tablespoon chopped fresh chives
1 tablespoon chopped fresh coriander
1 tablespoon cornflour
¼ cup water, extra
2 tablespoons evaporated skim milk

Boil, steam or microwave kumara and potatoes until tender, drain; place in bowl, mash well with fork. Mix in shallots and egg. Shape mixture into 8 patties, refrigerate 2 hours or until firm.

Heat oil in a frying pan, add potato cakes, cook until lightly browned on both sides, serve with sauce.

Fresh Herb Sauce: Combine water and stock cube in a small saucepan, add parsley, chives and coriander, bring to the boil, reduce heat, simmer 5 minutes. Blend cornflour with extra water, add to pan, stir constantly over heat until sauce boils and thickens. Stir in milk, heat without boiling.

Serves 4.

Approximately 835 kilojoules (200 calories) per serve.

HEARTY VEGETABLE LOAF

This recipe is not suitable to freeze or microwave.

2 cups coarsely grated carrot (240g)
1 cup coarsely grated potato (100g)
6 green shallots, chopped
1 small red pepper (100g)
2 small sticks celery (120g), chopped
1 cup stale wholemeal breadcrumbs
pinch cayenne pepper
2 eggs, lightly beaten
CHEESE SAUCE
30g butter
1 tablespoon plain flour
1 cup skim milk
¼ cup grated tasty cheese (30g)

Line an 11cm x 18cm loaf pan with foil. Combine all ingredients in bowl, mix well, press into loaf pan. Bake in moderate oven 50 minutes or until firm. Stand for 5 minutes before removing from pan, remove foil carefully, serve with sauce.

Cheese Sauce: Melt butter in a saucepan, stir in flour, cook 1 minute, stirring. Gradually stir in milk, stir constantly over heat until mixture boils and thickens, remove from heat, add cheese, stir until cheese is melted.

Serves 4.

Approximately 1030 kilojoules (246 calories) per serve.

ABOVE LEFT: Sweet Potato Cakes with Fresh Herb Sauce. ABOVE RIGHT: Hearty Vegetable Loaf. RIGHT: Pumpkin with Chilli Beans

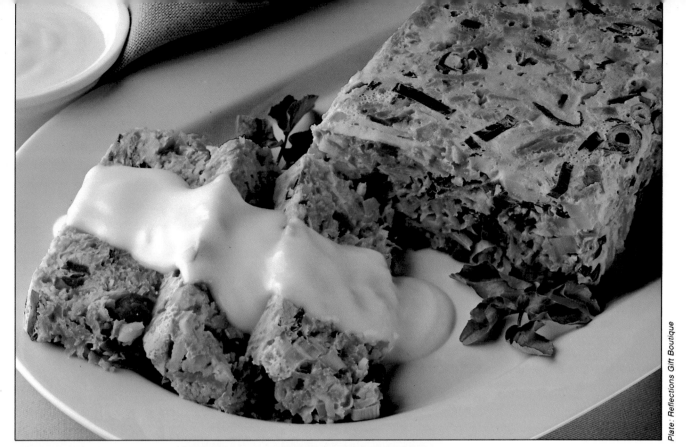

Plate: Reflections Gift Boutique

China: Villa Italiana; tiles: Country Floors

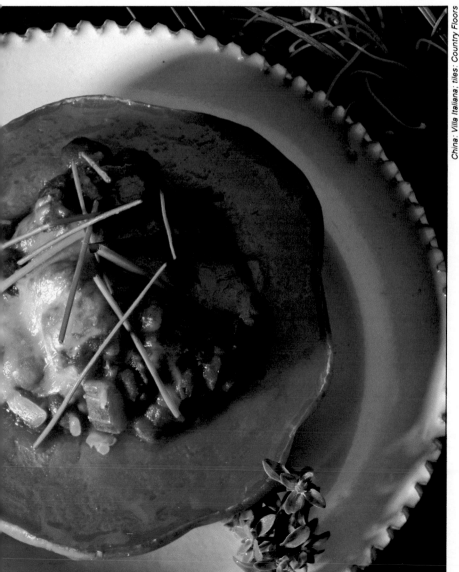

PUMPKIN WITH CHILLI BEANS

Bean topping can be prepared a day ahead. Recipe unsuitable to freeze.

1 butternut pumpkin (about 1kg)
¾ cup grated mozzarella cheese (90g)
TOPPING
1 medium onion (120g), finely chopped
2 teaspoons water
2 medium red peppers (300g), finely chopped
1 medium stick celery (80g), finely chopped
425g can tomatoes
310g can red kidney beans, rinsed, drained
1 tablespoon tomato sauce .
2 teaspoons Worcestershire sauce
pinch chilli powder

Cut pumpkin into 4 thick slices, remove seeds. Boil, steam or microwave pumpkin slices until just tender.

Place pumpkin slices on oven tray, divide topping evenly between slices, sprinkle with cheese. Bake in moderate oven for 10 minutes (or microwave on HIGH about 2 minutes).

Topping: Combine onion and water in saucepan, stir constantly over heat until onion is soft, add peppers and celery, stir over heat 2 minutes. Stir in undrained, crushed tomatoes, half the kidney beans, sauces and chilli powder. Mash remaining beans, add to saucepan, bring mixture to the boil, reduce heat, simmer, uncovered, until mixture is thick.

Serves 4.

Approximately 900 kilojoules (215 calories) per serve.

RABBIT

Rabbit is low in kilojoules and is almost fat free. It is readily obtainable from butchers, delicatessens and many chicken shops. It requires a moist method of cooking (such as being used in a casserole) to ensure tender meat with the best possible flavour.

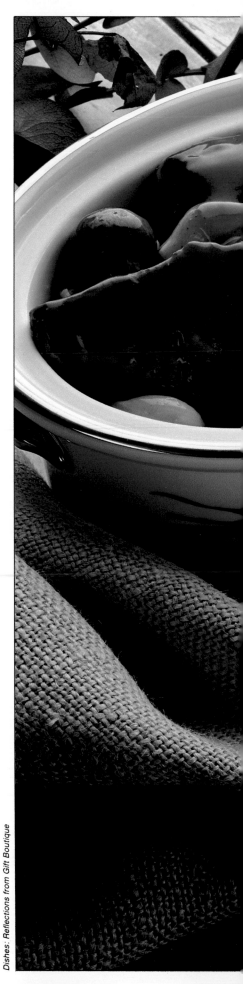

RABBIT, MUSHROOM AND RED WINE CASSEROLE

Golden shallots grow in clusters of up to 8 bulbs; the flavour is a subtle cross between onion and garlic. This recipe is not suitable to freeze.

4 x 200g rabbit pieces
125g golden shallots (10 large), peeled
½ cup dry red wine
1 tablespoon tomato paste
1 cup water
1 small chicken stock cube, crumbled
250g baby mushrooms
1 tablespoon cornflour
1 tablespoon water, extra

Place rabbit in an ovenproof dish; add whole shallots, red wine, tomato paste, water and stock cube, cover, bake in moderate oven for about 1 hour (or microwave on MEDIUM for about 30 minutes). Add mushrooms, bake further 30 minutes (or microwave on HIGH about 10 minutes) or until rabbit is tender. Remove rabbit and vegetables from dish, keep warm.

Strain liquid into saucepan, add blended cornflour and extra water into pan, stir constantly over heat until mixture boils and thickens. Place rabbit and vegetables in serving dish, pour sauce over rabbit.

Serves 4.

Approximately 835 kilojoules (199 calories) per serve.

HEARTY RABBIT AND TOMATO CASSEROLE

This recipe can be frozen for up to 2 months.

2 teaspoons oil
4 x 200g rabbit pieces
½ cup dry red wine
2 medium tomatoes (200g), chopped
1 medium carrot (120g), sliced
2 teaspoons grated orange rind
1 bay leaf
1 teaspoon dried oregano leaves
2 teaspoons white vinegar
1 small chicken stock cube, crumbled
1 cup water
2 teaspoons cornflour
¼ cup water, extra

Heat oil in a frying pan, add rabbit, cook, turning, until lightly browned all over. Place rabbit in an ovenproof dish.

Add wine to pan, cook, stirring, for 1 minute, pour wine over rabbit. Add tomatoes, carrot, rind, bay leaf, oregano, vinegar, stock cube and water to dish, cover, bake in moderate oven for about 1½ hours (or microwave on MEDIUM for about 40 minutes) or until rabbit is tender. Remove rabbit from dish, keep warm.

Pour vegetable mixture into a saucepan, stir in blended cornflour and extra water, stir constantly over heat until mixture boils and thickens (or microwave on HIGH for about 3 minutes). Place rabbit in serving dish, pour sauce over rabbit.

Serves 4.

Approximately 830 kilojoules (198 calories) per serve.

Top: Rabbit, Mushroom and Red Wine Casserole; bottom: Hearty Rabbit and Tomato Casserole

Dishes: Reflections from Gift Boutique

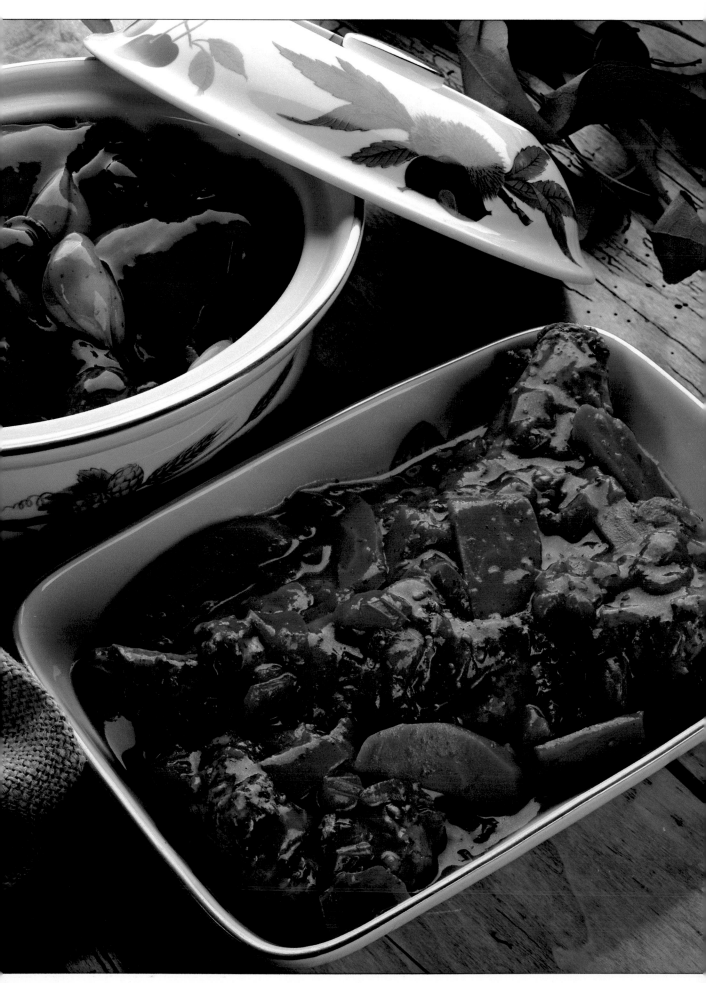

KILOJOULE & CALORIE COUNTER

		kJ	cal
Abalone:	uncooked, 100g	410	98
	cooked, 100g	605	145
Alfalfa sprouts:	20g = ½ cup	25	6
All-bran:	1 cup = 60g	860	205
Almonds:	flaked, slivered, ¼ cup = 25g	585	140
	ground, 1 tablespoon = 10g	235	56
	blanched, kernels, ¼ cup = 45g	1050	251
Anchovies:	1 canned, drained	35	8
Apple:	fresh, large, 200g	300	72
	dried, whole, ½ cup = 100g	1210	289
	juice, ¼ cup	120	29
	sauce, ¼ cup	105	25
Apricots:	fresh, dried, unsweetened		
	canned	85	20
	glacé	410	98
	nectar, ¼ cup	165	39
Arrowroot:	1 teaspoon	40	10
Artichoke:	raw, medium, 375g	120	28
	canned heart in brine	40	10
Asparagus:	canned cuts, drained, ½ cup	65	16
	raw or canned, drained, 6 spears	60	14
Avocado:	fresh, medium, 200g	1640	392
Bacon rasher:	uncooked, medium, 40g	700	167
	grilled	420	100
Baking powder:	1 teaspoon	15	4
Bamboo shoots:	raw, 40g piece	45	11
	canned, drained, ½ cup	35	8
Banana (with skin):	fresh, medium, 150g	370	88
Barbecue sauce:	1 tablespoon	110	26

		kJ	cal
Barley:	raw, ½ cup = 100g	1535	367
	cooked, ½ cup	435	104
Beans:	baked in tomato sauce, ⅓ cup = 100g	270	65
	broad, shelled, cooked, ½ cup = 75g	205	49
	dried (eg. kidney, soy) cooked (or canned), ½ cup = 100g	400	96
	green, canned, fresh or frozen, ¾ cup chopped = 100g	30	7
	green, dehydrated, 1 cup = 50g	150	36
Bean sprouts:	½ cup = 30g	30	7
Beef consommé:	canned, ½ cup	70	17
Beef:	uncooked blade steak, 250g	1365	326
	uncooked chuck steak, 250g	1140	272
	uncooked eye fillet, 250g	1305	312
	uncooked lean minced, 250g	1845	440
	uncooked round steak, 250g	1340	320
	uncooked rump, 250g	1105	264
	uncooked sausage, 1 thick	1240	296
	cooked	830	198
	uncooked sausage, 1 thin	870	208
	cooked	610	146
	uncooked scotch fillet, 250g	1390	332
	uncooked sirloin, 250g	1550	370
	uncooked T-bone, 250g	1315	314
	uncooked topside, 250g	1250	299
Beer:	375ml can	650	155
	375ml can, low alcohol	400	96
	375ml can, special light (0.9 percent alcohol)	300	72
Beetroot:	raw, medium, 160g	190	45

This kilojoule/calorie counter has been compiled by nutritionist Rosemary Stanton using the most up to date information available. The calories have been calculated by dividing the number of kilojoules by 4·186, then adjusting to the nearest practical number. The counts have been estimated on the bought weights to help you work out your shopping list.

The meat is estimated on lean cuts, the fruit and vegetables mainly on average-sized items. The kilojoule count does change in some food after it has been cooked, we have included both counts where appropriate.

Fat and oil-free methods of cooking were used, such as grilling, poaching, steaming, microwaving and boiling. Quantities estimated in this counter were calculated using metric measuring spoons and cups. To help you adjust amounts of ingredients, it is handy to know that there are 4 teaspoons in one tablespoon and there are 12 tablespoons in one cup.

		kJ	cal
Beetroot:	cooked, ½ cup	190	45
	canned, drained, 100g	140	33
Biscuit crumbs:	sweet, 1 cup = 125g	2240	535
Black beans:	canned or dried, 1 tablespoon	275	66
Black bean sauce:	1 tablespoon	170	40
Blackberries:	fresh, ½ punnet = 125g	155	37
	canned in syrup, drained, ½ cup	375	90
Black pudding:	100g	1080	258
Blueberries:	fresh, ½ punnet = 125g	295	70
	canned in syrup, drained, ½ cup	460	110
Boysenberries:	fresh, ½ punnet = 125g	185	44
	canned in syrup, drained, ½ cup	405	97
Brains:	uncooked, 1 set = 100g	505	121
	cooked, 100g	565	135
Bran flakes:	1 cup = 45g	685	164
Bran:	unprocessed, 1 tablespoon	65	16
Brazil nut kernels:	¼ cup = 40g	1020	244
Bread:	any type, 1 slice	270	65
	any type, 1 toast (thick) slice	420	100
	crumbs, packaged, ½ cup = 50g	755	180
	stale, ½ cup = 35g	395	94
	roll, large	630	150
	roll, small	385	92
Broccoli:	raw, 100g	95	23
	cooked, 100g	80	19
Brussels sprouts:	raw, 100g	110	26
	cooked, 100g	75	18
Buckwheat:	1 tablespoon	270	65

		kJ	cal
Burghul (cracked wheat):	soaked, drained, ½ cup	460	110
Butter:	1 tablespoon	615	147
Buttermilk:	250ml	470	112
Cabanossi:	50g	760	182
Cabbage:	raw, 1 cup shredded = 80g	90	22
	cooked, ½ cup	40	10
	Chinese, 1 cup shredded = 50g	35	8
	cooked, ½ cup	50	12
	red, 1 cup shredded = 80g	70	17
	cooked, ½ cup	65	16
Cannelloni (pasta):	1 tube cooked	125	30
Carob powder:	1 tablespoon	150	36
Carrot:	raw, medium, 120g	125	30
	cooked, ½ cup	85	20
	440g can, drained	360	86
Cashews:	⅓ cup = 50g	1200	287
Cauliflower:	raw, 100g	55	13
	cooked, 100g	40	10
Caviar:	lumpfish roe, 1 tablespoon	175	42
Celery:	raw, medium stick, 80g	30	7
	cooked, ½ cup	20	5
Cheese:	blue vein, 30g	440	105
	brie, 30g	400	96
	camembert, 30g	375	90
	cheddar, processed, 30g	400	96
	cottage, 30g	115	27
	cotto, low-fat, 30g	270	65
	cream, 30g	430	103
	edam, 30g	380	91
	emmenthal, 30g	460	110

		kJ	cal
Cheese:	fetta, 30g	380	91
	gorgonzola, 30g	460	110
	gouda, 30g	480	115
	gruyere, 30g	460	110
	havarti, 30g	535	128
	Jarlsberg, 30g	375	90
	mascarpone, 30g	430	103
	mozzarella, 30g	380	91
	parmesan, grated (1 tablespoon)	170	41
	ricotta, 30g	190	45
	stilton, 30g	575	137
	Swiss, 30g	460	110
	tasty cheddar, 30g (¼ cup grated)	505	121
Cherries:	fresh, ¾ cup = 125g	250	60
	canned, sweetened, drained, ½ cup	435	104
	whole, glacé, ½ cup = 110g	1565	374
Chicken (all cuts without skin):	uncooked, 115g breast fillet	540	129
	cooked, 100g	660	158
	uncooked, 85g drumstick	450	108
	uncooked, 75g thigh fillet	400	96
	uncooked, 200g chicken breast on the bone	770	184
	uncooked, 100g chicken wing	310	74
	uncooked, 375g chicken maryland	1150	275
Chicken stock cube:	small	15	4
Chick peas:	raw, ½ cup = 100g	1360	325
	cooked, ½ cup	600	143
Chicory (witlof):	raw, 50g	30	7
Chilli sauce:	1 teaspoon	10	2
Chocolate:	100g	2250	538
Choko:	raw, medium, 100g	115	27
	cooked, ½ cup	105	25
Chutney:	1 tablespoon	160	38
Cocoa powder:	1 teaspoon	35	8
Coconut:	desiccated, 1 tablespoon	185	44
	flaked or shredded, ¼ cup	375	90
	fresh, 50g piece	725	173
	canned cream, ½ cup	1260	301
	canned milk, ¼ cup	515	123
Cod (smoked):	150g	500	119
Copha:	1 tablespoon	670	160
Corn:	1 cob = 275g	485	116
	½ cup, kernels cooked	285	68
	canned kernels, ¼ cup	140	33
	creamed, ¼ cup	170	41
	425g can baby whole corn, drained	375	90
Corn relish:	1 tablespoon	85	20
Corned beef:	cooked, 100g	805	192
Cornflakes:	1 cup = 30g	475	113
Cornflour:	1 tablespoon	150	36
Corn syrup:	1 tablespoon	210	50
Crab:	100g flesh	420	100
	170g can, drained	580	139

		kJ	cal
Crayfish (lobster):	medium tail = 100g flesh	395	94
Cream:	fresh (thick and pouring), 1 tablespoon	285	68
	reduced (canned), 1 tablespoon	225	54
	sour (commercial), 1 tablespoon	280	67
	sour light (commercial), 1 tablespoon	165	39
Croissant:	1 medium	1000	239
Crumpet:	1 medium	400	96
Cucumber:	raw, medium, 280g	120	29
Cumquats:	fresh, 100g	200	48
Currants:	fresh, red/black, 100g	90	22
	dried, ½ cup = 70g	725	173
Curry powder:	1 teaspoon	25	6
Custard apple:	fresh, 100g	310	74
Custard powder:	1 tablespoon	150	36
Cuttlefish:	uncooked, 100g	290	69
Dates:	dried, ½ cup chopped = 90g	950	227
	fresh, 2 = 30g	60	14
Dressing:	refer to Glossary and individual brands of commercial dressings		
Duck:	uncooked, 100g, without skin	515	123
	roasted, with skin, 100g	1405	336
	roasted, without skin, 100g	790	189
Egg:	small (45g)	250	60
	medium (55g)	300	72
	large (61g)	335	80
	small egg yolk	205	49
	small egg white	45	11
	medium egg yolk	250	60
	medium egg white	50	12
	large egg yolk	275	66
	large egg white	60	14
Egg noodles:	raw, 100g	1620	387
	cooked, ½ cup	420	100
Eel:	uncooked, 100g	700	167
	cooked, 100g	840	201
Eggplant:	raw, medium, 320g	200	48
	cooked, 100g	80	19
Endive:	raw, 1 leaf = 30g	15	4
English spinach:	raw, 20 leaves = 100g	80	19
	cooked, ½ cup	130	31
Evaporated milk:	1 tablespoon	125	30
	½ cup	770	184
Evaporated skim milk: (0.5% fat)	1 tablespoon	60	14
	½ cup	420	100
Fennel:	raw, medium bulb = 300g	85	20
Fettuccine (pasta):	raw, 100g	1575	376
	cooked, ½ cup	355	85
Fig:	fresh, medium, 85g	145	35
	dried, 100g	910	217
Fillo pastry:	1 sheet	105	25
Fish:	uncooked, white (non-oily) 125g fillet (see Glossary)	485	116

		kJ	cal
Fish:	cooked, 100g	425	102
Flour (all types):	1 tablespoon	185	44
	½ cup = 75g	1130	270
Frankfurt:	1 large = 85g	965	230
Garlic:	1 clove	15	4
Gelatine:	1 teaspoon	40	10
Ghee:	1 tablespoon	695	166
Gherkin:	medium, 30g	65	15
Ginger:	fresh, 1 teaspoon grated	10	2
	crystallised and glacé, 1 tablespoon finely chopped = 20g	285	68
Glucose syrup:	1 tablespoon	270	65
Goats' milk:	250ml	740	177
Golden syrup:	1 teaspoon	60	14
Grapefruit:	fresh, medium, 390g	175	42
	juice, ¼ cup	95	23
Grapes:	fresh, 250g	710	170
	juice = ¼ cup	215	51
Guava:	fresh, medium, 115g	115	27
Haddock:	smoked, 150g	645	154
Ham:	30g slice	150	36
Hazelnuts:	roasted kernels, ¼ cup = 45g	705	168
	ground, 1 tablespoon = 10g	155	37
Heart:	uncooked, 125g ox	530	127
	cooked, 100g	625	149
	uncooked, 125g sheep	640	153
	cooked, 100g	770	184
Herbs:	dried leaves, 1 teaspoon	20	5
	fresh, chopped, 1 teaspoon	5	1
Honey:	1 teaspoon	65	16
	1 tablespoon	270	65
Honeydew melon:	fresh, medium, 1250g	700	167
Ice-cream:	10 percent fat, ½ cup serve	575	137
	rich, 16 percent fat, ½ cup serve	950	227
	tofu, 8 percent fat, ½ cup serve	660	158
	low kilojoule, no fat, ½ cup serve	250	60
Jam:	1 teaspoon	55	13
	low kilojoule, 1 teaspoon	10	2
Jelly:	½ cup	390	93
	low kilojoule, ½ cup	40	10
Kidneys:	uncooked, lambs, 2 = 100g	385	92
	cooked, 100g	610	146
Kiwi fruit:	fresh, medium, 100g	175	40
Kohlrabi:	raw, medium, 300g	365	87
	cooked, ½ cup	100	24
Kumara:	raw, medium, 300g	1020	244
	cooked, ½ cup	340	81
Lamb:	uncooked, 1 chump chop = 150g	885	211
	uncooked, 1 small cutlet =75g	450	108
	uncooked, 1 loin chop = 100g	530	127

		kJ	cal
Lamb:	uncooked, 1 shank = 300g	2230	533
Lasagne (pasta):	uncooked, 1 sheet	215	51
Lecithin granules:	1 tablespoon	315	75
Leek:	raw, medium, 200g	255	61
	cooked, sliced, ½ cup	105	25
Lemon:	fresh, medium, 180g	115	27
	juice, ¼ cup	20	5
Lentils:	raw, ⅔ cup = 100g	1295	310
	cooked, ½ cup	420	100
Lettuce:	raw (all types), 2 medium leaves	20	5
Lime:	fresh, medium, 85g	80	19
	juice, ¼ cup	65	16
Liqueurs (all types):	1 tablespoon	250	60
Liver:	uncooked, calf, 60g	350	84
	cooked, 100g	745	178
	uncooked, chicken, 60g	340	81
	uncooked, duck, 60g	420	100
	uncooked, lamb, 60g	410	98
	cooked, 100g	1010	241
Liverwurst:	50g	655	156
Lobster (crayfish):	uncooked, medium tail = 100g flesh	395	94
Loganberries:	fresh, ½ punnet = 125g	305	73
	canned in syrup, drained, ½ cup	535	128
Loquat:	fresh, medium, 20g	15	4
Lychees:	fresh, 5 medium, 115g	225	54
	canned in syrup, drained, ½ cup	270	65
Macadamia nuts:	whole, ¼ cup = 45g	1330	318
Macaroni:	raw, 1 cup = 100g	1575	376
	cooked, ½ cup	355	85
Madeira:	1 tablespoon	120	29
Malted milk powder:	1 tablespoon	255	61
Malt extract:	1 tablespoon	375	90
Mandarin:	fresh, medium, 105g	200	48
Mango:	fresh, medium, 240g	425	102
	canned in syrup, drained, ½ cup	420	100
Margarine:	1 tablespoon	615	147
Marmalade:	1 teaspoon	55	13
Marrow:	raw, 100g	70	17
	cooked, ½ cup	30	7
Marsala:	1 tablespoon	155	37
Mayonnaise:	1 tablespoon	630	150
	low oil, 1 tablespoon	165	39
Milk:	250ml whole, 3.8 percent fat	725	173
	250ml skim, 0.1 percent fat	355	85
	250ml evaporated, 8 percent fat	1570	375
	250ml evaporated skim, 0.5 percent fat	835	199
Milk powder:	full cream, 1 tablespoon	215	51
	skim, 1 tablespoon	150	36
Mint jelly:	1 teaspoon	65	16
Mixed peel:	½ cup = 110g	1285	307
Moreton Bay bugs:	uncooked, 100g flesh	385	92
Mortadella:	4 slices = 60g	815	195
Muesli:	natural, ½ cup = 50g	775	185

		kJ	cal
Muesli:	toasted, ½ cup = 50g	935	223
Mulberries:	fresh, ½ punnet = 125g	190	45
Mushrooms:	raw, 100g	55	13
	canned whole (champignons) drained, ½ cup = 100g	70	17
	Chinese, dried, 6 whole	60	14
	oyster (abalone), 100g	75	18
Mussels:	uncooked, 6 medium	220	53
Mustard:	1 teaspoon	25	6
Nectarine:	fresh, large, 180g	355	85
Noodles:	raw, 100g	1575	376
	cooked, ½ cup	355	85
Oats:	raw, 1 cup = 100g	1545	369
	cooked, ½ cup	225	54
Octopus:	uncooked, medium, 200g	570	136
Okra:	raw, 250g	180	43
	cooked, ½ cup	45	11
Oil (all types):	1 teaspoon	185	44
Olives:	6 black	255	60
	6 green	150	36
Onion:	raw, medium, 120g	120	29
	small, pickled	50	12
Orange:	fresh, large, 220g	250	60
	juice, ¼ cup	115	28
Oysters:	uncooked, 6 medium	130	31
	smoked, canned, 6 medium	550	131
Oyster sauce:	1 teaspoon	25	6
Parsley:	fresh, 1 tablespoon, chopped	5	1
Parsnip:	raw, medium, 200g	420	100
	cooked, ½ cup	240	57
Passionfruit:	medium, 55g	45	11
Pasta (all types):	uncooked, 100g	1575	376
	cooked, ½ cup	355	85
Pawpaw:	fresh, 1 medium, 1500g	1645	393
	½ cup, chopped, dried = 105g	115	27
Peach:	fresh, or unsweetened canned, drained, 150g	205	49
	canned in syrup, 2 halves	450	108
	glacé, 35g	440	105
	dried, ½ cup = 80g	725	173
	nectar, ¼ cup	115	27
Peanuts:	roasted, ¼ cup = 40g	945	226
Peanut butter:	1 teaspoon	130	31
Pear:	fresh, medium, 150g	250	60
	canned in syrup, drained, 2 halves	410	98
	dried, 30g	240	57
	glacé, 30g	375	90
	juice, ¼ cup	135	32
Peas:	raw or frozen, ½ cup	140	33
	canned, ½ cup drained	200	48
Pecans:	¼ cup kernels = 25g	630	150
Pepino:	fresh, medium, 135g	115	28
Pepper (capsicum):	raw, medium, 150g	100	24
	cooked, 100g	60	14

		kJ	cal
Persimmon:	fresh, medium, 115g	215	51
Pickles:	1 tablespoon	105	25
Pimiento:	canned or bottled, 1 whole pepper, drained = 60g	55	13
Pineapple:	fresh or unsweetened canned, 3 x 1cm slices = 150g	245	59
	sweetened, canned, drained, 1 slice	375	90
	unsweetened juice, ¼ cup	115	27
Pine nuts:	¼ cup = 45g	970	232
Pistachio nuts:	shelled, ¼ cup = 40g	970	232
Plum:	fresh, medium, 70g	110	26
	canned in syrup, drained, ½ cup	435	104
Pomegranate:	fresh, large, 460g	730	174
Poppy seeds:	1 teaspoon	65	16
Pork:	uncooked, butterfly steak, 175g	790	189
	uncooked, fillet, 100g	435	104
	uncooked, loin chop, 190g	425	102
	uncooked, sausage, 1 thick	1520	363
	cooked	925	221
	uncooked, sausage, 1 thin	1065	254
	cooked	660	158
	uncooked, steak, 100g	430	103
Port:	1 tablespoon	130	31
Potato:	raw, medium, 100g	360	86
	cooked, 100g	330	79
	crisps, 25g packet	545	130
Prawns:	uncooked, medium, 250g in shells	430	103
	shelled, cooked, 100g	450	108
Prickly pear:	fresh, medium, 110g	135	32
Prosciutto:	50g	270	64
Prunes (dried plums):	½ cup = 65g	445	106
Puff pastry:	1 sheet ready rolled, cooked	2715	649
Pumpernickel:	1 slice, 30g	300	72
Pumpkin (all types):	raw, 500g with skin and seeds	245	59
	cooked, ½ cup	65	16
	seed kernels (pepitas), 1 tablespoon = 12g	235	56
Quail:	uncooked, 150g	745	178
Quince:	fresh, medium, 220g	235	56
Rabbit:	uncooked, 200g	1040	248
	cooked, 100g	750	179
Radish:	raw, medium	10	2
Raisins:	½ cup = 80g	840	200
Raisin bread:	toast (thick) slice	275	66
Raspberries:	fresh, ½ punnet = 125g	130	31
	canned in syrup, drained, ½ cup	460	110
Rhubarb:	fresh or frozen, chopped, 1 cup = 85g	22	5
	cooked, 1 cup sweetened	380	90
Rice (all types):	raw, ½ cup = 100g	1530	365
	½ cup boiled or steamed	670	160
Rice Bubbles:	1 cup = 30g	475	113
Rice flour:	ground rice, 1 tablespoon	305	73

		kJ	cal
Rockmelon:	fresh, medium, 1750g	1100	263
Sago:	raw, ½ cup = 100g	1515	362
	cooked, ½ cup	380	91
Salami:	50g	900	215
	Polish 50g	505	121
Salmon:	uncooked, 125g fillet	735	176
	210g can, drained	1365	326
	smoked, 30g	180	43
Sardines:	uncooked, medium, 100g	420	100
	110g can in oil, drained	960	229
Satay sauce:	1 teaspoon	65	16
Scallops (Tasmanian):	uncooked, 250g	860	205
Semolina:	raw, ½ cup = 100g	1490	356
	cooked, ½ cup	370	88
Sesame oil:	1 teaspoon	185	44
Sesame seeds:	1 teaspoon	60	14
Shallots:	golden, medium = 15g	45	11
	green, 6 medium	90	22
Sherry:	dry, 1 tablespoon	95	23
	sweet, 1 tablespoon	115	27
	after heating	15	4
Silver beet (spinach):	raw, 5 medium leaves = 100g	115	27
	cooked, ½ cup	125	30
Snow peas:	raw, 100g	160	38
Soya sauce:	1 teaspoon	15	4
Spaghetti (pasta):	raw, 100g	1575	376
	cooked, ½ cup	355	85
Spices, ground:	1 teaspoon	30	7
Spinach (English):	raw, 20 leaves = 100g	80	19
	cooked, ½ cup	130	31
(silver beet)	5 medium leaves = 100g	115	27
Spirits (including rum, whisky, gin):	1 tablespoon	195	47
Split peas:	cooked, ½ cup	405	97
Spring onion:	raw, medium, 40g	60	14
Squash:	raw, 250g	200	48
	cooked, ½ cup	60	14
Squid:	uncooked, 250g	785	188
Stock cube:	small (or 1 teaspoon bouillon powder)	20	5
Stout:	375ml	600	143
Strawberries:	fresh, ½ punnet = 125g	135	32
	canned in syrup, drained, ½ cup	430	103
Sugar, (all types):	1 teaspoon	80	19
	½ cup	2040	487
Sultanas:	½ cup = 80g	855	204
Sunflower seed kernels:	1 tablespoon = 15g	480	115
Swede:	raw, medium, 300g	265	63
	cooked, ½ cup	75	18
Sweetened condensed milk:	1 tablespoon	360	86
	skim, 1 tablespoon	295	70
Sweet potato:	raw, medium, 375g	1450	346
	cooked, ½ cup	365	87

		kJ	cal
Tacos:	1 medium	210	50
Tahini:	1 teaspoon	120	29
Tamarillo:	fresh, medium, 75g	80	19
Tangelo:	fresh, medium, 170g	165	39
Tangerine:	fresh, medium, 190g	195	47
Teriyaki sauce:	1 teaspoon	20	5
Tofu:	100g	290	69
Tomato:	fresh, medium, 100g	90	22
	canned, drained, ½ cup	70	17
	juice, ¼ cup	60	14
	paste, 1 teaspoon	20	5
	purée, ¼ cup	105	25
	sauce, 1 tablespoon	65	16
Tongue:	uncooked, 100g	835	199
	cooked, 100g	1290	308
Tripe:	uncooked, 100g	300	72
	cooked, 100g	350	84
Tuna:	uncooked, 125g fillet	635	152
	185g canned in brine, drained	815	195
	185g canned in oil, drained	1325	317
Turkey:	uncooked, 125g fillet	570	136
	cooked, 100g	595	142
Turnip:	raw, medium, 200g	170	41
	cooked, ½ cup	50	12
Veal:	uncooked, chop/cutlet, 125g	470	112
	uncooked, steak/schnitzel, 125g	545	130
Vegemite, Marmite; Promite:	½ teaspoon	20	5
Vegeroni:	raw, 1¼ cups = 100g	400	95
	cooked, ½ cup	225	54
Venison:	uncooked, 125g	660	158
	cooked	630	150
Vermouth:	dry, 1 tablespoon	100	24
	sweet, 1 tablespoon	125	30
Vinegar:	brown or white, 1 tablespoon	5	1
Vine leaves:	fresh or packaged, 200g	160	38
Walnuts:	¼ cup chopped = 30g	650	155
Water chestnuts:	canned, drained, ½ cup	215	51
Water crackers:	10 small = 40g	745	178
Watercress:	raw, 1 cup leaves = 30g	20	5
Watermelon:	fresh, 1 cup chopped flesh = 250g	250	60
Wheatgerm:	1 tablespoon	125	30
Wild rice:	raw, ½ cup = 100g	1480	354
	cooked, ½ cup	330	79
Wine:	red or white, ¼ cup	230	55
	when used in cooking	0	0
Witlof (chicory):	raw, 50g	30	7
Worcestershire sauce:	1 teaspoon	25	6
Yoghurt:	natural, 200g carton	645	154
	low-fat plain, 200g carton	500	119
Zucchini:	raw, medium, 150g	90	22
	cooked, ½ cup	60	14

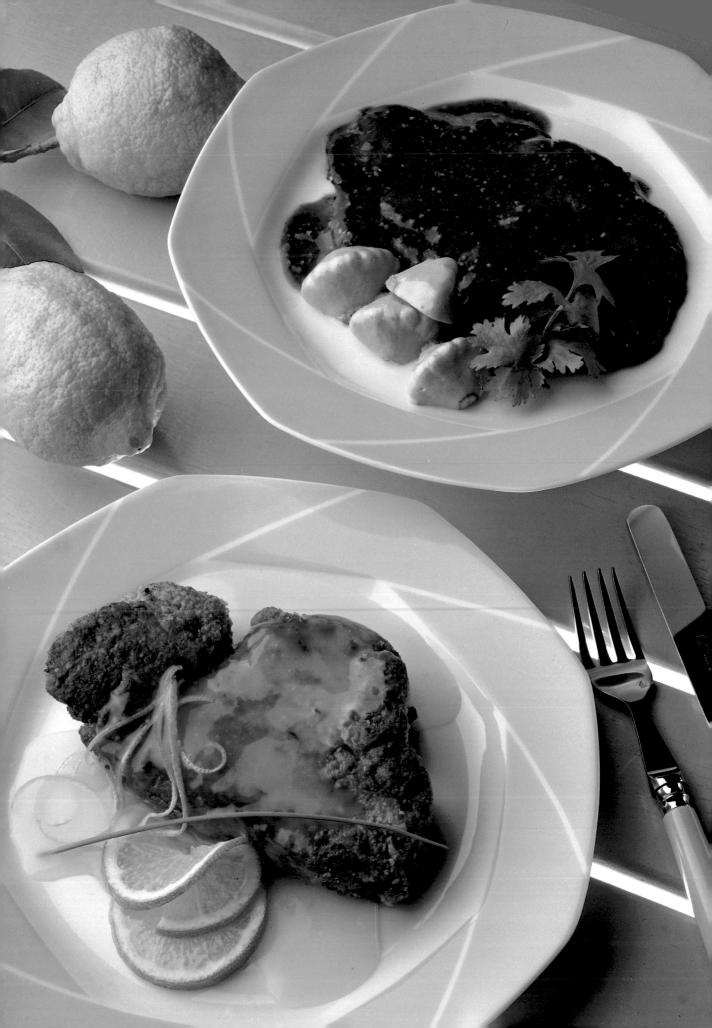

Try using some of our superb sauces and glazes to enhance the delicate flavour of veal. This meat is lean even without trimming. If using veal steaks, remove the membrane before cooking, otherwise steaks will curl.

MUSTARD GLAZED VEAL

This recipe is not suitable to freeze or microwave.

2 tablespoons tomato sauce
2 teaspoons Worcestershire sauce
1 tablespoon seeded mustard
1 tablespoon brown sugar
1 tablespoon white vinegar
4 x 100g veal steaks
1 teaspoon cornflour
¼ cup water

Combine sauces, mustard, sugar and vinegar in bowl, add steaks, mix well to coat with mixture, cover, refrigerate several hours or overnight.

Remove steaks from mustard mixture, reserve mustard mixture, place steaks into heated frying pan, cook until tender and browned all over. Remove steaks from pan; keep warm. Drain any liquid from pan, blend cornflour and water into remaining mustard mixture, add to pan, stir constantly over heat until mixture boils and thickens. Spoon glaze over steaks.
Serves 4.

■ *Approximately 550 kilojoules (131 calories) per serve.*

VEAL STEAKS WITH FRESH ASPARAGUS SPEARS

This recipe is not suitable to freeze or microwave.

12 asparagus spears
2 teaspoons oil
4 x 100g veal steaks
¼ teaspoon dried thyme leaves
½ small beef stock cube, crumbled
½ cup water
1 tablespoon cornflour
¾ cup water, extra
¼ cup dry red wine

Trim asparagus with a vegetable peeler. Heat oil in frying pan, add steaks and thyme, cook on both sides until browned and steaks are tender, remove from pan, keep warm. Add stock cube and water to pan, bring to the boil, add asparagus, reduce heat, simmer 2 minutes, remove from pan. Return stock to the boil, add blended cornflour, extra water and wine, stir constantly over heat until mixture boils and thickens. Serve veal with sauce and asparagus.
Serves 4.

■ *Approximately 520 kilojoules (124 calories) per serve.*

CRUMBED VEAL CHOPS WITH CITRUS SAUCE

Veal can be crumbed up to 12 hours ahead. This recipe is not suitable to freeze or microwave.

16 small water crackers (70g)
1 teaspoon grated lemon or lime rind
4 x 125g veal chops
1 egg, lightly beaten
1 tablespoon water
1½ tablespoons oil
CITRUS SAUCE
2 teaspoons cornflour
¾ cup water
2 tablespoons lemon or lime juice
½ small chicken stock cube, crumbled
1 teaspoon sugar

Blend or process crackers until fine. Mix rind into crumbs. Toss chops into crumbs, dip into combined egg and water then toss in crumbs again; refrigerate 30 minutes before cooking.

Heat oil in frying pan, add chops, cook until browned on both sides. Place chops onto oven tray, bake in moderate oven for about 45 minutes or until tender. Serve chops with sauce.
Citrus Sauce: Blend cornflour with water in saucepan, add remaining ingredients, stir constantly over heat until mixture boils and thickens (or microwave on HIGH about 1 minute).
Serves 4.

■ *Approximately 1195 kilojoules (285 calories) per serve.*

APRICOT CORIANDER VEAL

This recipe is not suitable to freeze or microwave.

4 x 100g veal steaks
2 teaspoons ground coriander
2 tablespoons plain flour
1 tablespoon oil
½ cup apricot nectar
1 small chicken stock cube, crumbled
½ cup water

Toss veal in combined coriander and flour, shake away excess flour mixture. Heat oil in frying pan, add veal, cook over high heat until browned on both sides; drain on absorbent paper.

Add apricot nectar, stock cube and water to pan, bring to the boil, boil 2 minutes. Return veal to pan, reduce heat, simmer, covered, 10 minutes or until veal is tender.
Serves 4.

■ *Approximately 730 kilojoules (174 calories) per serve.*

BELOW: Veal Steaks with Fresh Asparagus Spears. OPPOSITE PAGE: Top: Mustard Glazed Veal; bottom: Crumbed Veal Chops with Citrus Sauce

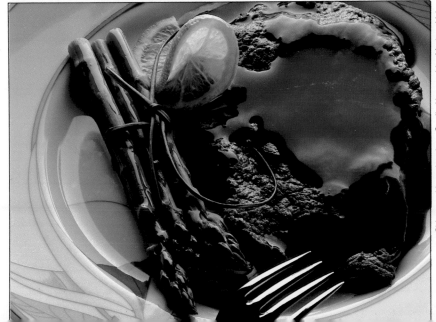

VEAL CUTLETS PAPRIKA

This dish can be frozen for up to 2 months.

1 teaspoon oil
1 medium onion (120g), sliced
1 clove garlic, crushed
4 x 125g veal cutlets
1 teaspoon paprika
2 teaspoons plain flour
1 teaspoon oil, extra
2 tablespoons tomato paste
2 tablespoons dry red wine
1 small chicken stock cube,
**   crumbled**
1 cup water

Heat oil in a frying pan, add onion and garlic, cook, stirring constantly, until onion is soft; remove from pan.

Lightly dust cutlets in combined paprika and flour, reserve flour. Heat extra oil in pan, add cutlets, cook over high heat until browned on both sides, place into ovenproof dish. Add remaining flour mixture to pan, stir in tomato paste, wine, stock cube and water. Stir constantly over heat until mixture boils and thickens, add onion; pour mixture over cutlets.

Cover, bake in moderate oven about 25 minutes (or microwave on HIGH about 7 minutes) or until tender. Serves 4.

Approximately 670 kilojoules (160 calories) per serve.

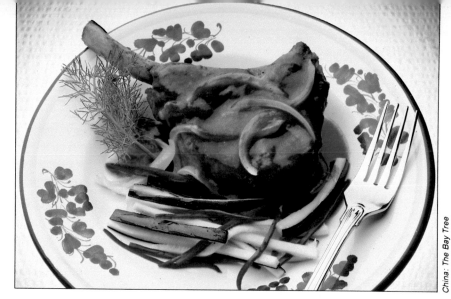

China: Studio Haus

CREAMY VEAL WITH MUSHROOM SAUCE

Unsuitable to freeze or microwave.

4 x 100g veal steaks
2 teaspoons oil
125g mushrooms, thinly sliced
3 green shallots, finely chopped
½ cup dry white wine
⅓ cup unsweetened tomato juice
1½ tablespoons sour light cream
1 small beef stock cube, crumbled
½ teaspoon sugar

Pound steaks thinly with meat mallet. Heat oil in frying pan, add steaks, cook until tender and well browned all over; remove steaks from pan, keep warm.

Add mushrooms and shallots to pan, stir constantly over heat until mushrooms are tender. Stir in wine, bring to the boil, boil, uncovered, for 2 minutes. Stir in tomato juice, cream, stock cube and sugar. Return steaks to pan, simmer, uncovered, 2 minutes. Serves 4.

Approximately 580 kilojoules (138 calories) per serve.

TASTY VEAL PARCELS

Recipe unsuitable to freeze.

4 x 100g veal steaks
1 small carrot (80g)
125g mushrooms, sliced
1 teaspoon light soya sauce
½ teaspoon dried marjoram leaves
2 teaspoons tomato paste
½ cup water
1 small chicken stock cube, crumbled
¼ cup evaporated skim milk

Pound steaks thinly with meat mallet. Cut carrot into thin strips. Place carrot, mushrooms, soya sauce, marjoram, tomato paste, water and stock cube into a frying pan, bring to the boil, reduce heat, simmer for 3 minutes (or microwave on HIGH for 2 minutes). Strain mixture, reserve liquid.

Divide vegetable mixture between steaks, fold in sides, roll up into parcels; tie with string. Return reserved liquid to pan, reheat, add veal parcels, simmer for about 10 minutes (or microwave on HIGH for about 8 minutes) or until tender. Remove parcels from pan, keep warm.

Add evaporated milk to liquid in pan, heat without boiling (or microwave on HIGH for about 1 minute). Remove string from veal parcels. Cut parcels into slices. Serve with sauce. Serves 4.

Approximately 475 kilojoules (113 calories) per serve.

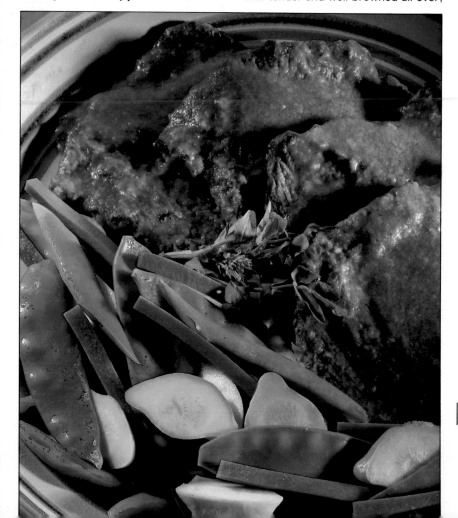

LEFT: Apricot Coriander Veal. ABOVE: Veal Cutlets Paprika. RIGHT: Top: Tasty Veal Parcels; bottom: Creamy Veal with Mushroom Sauce

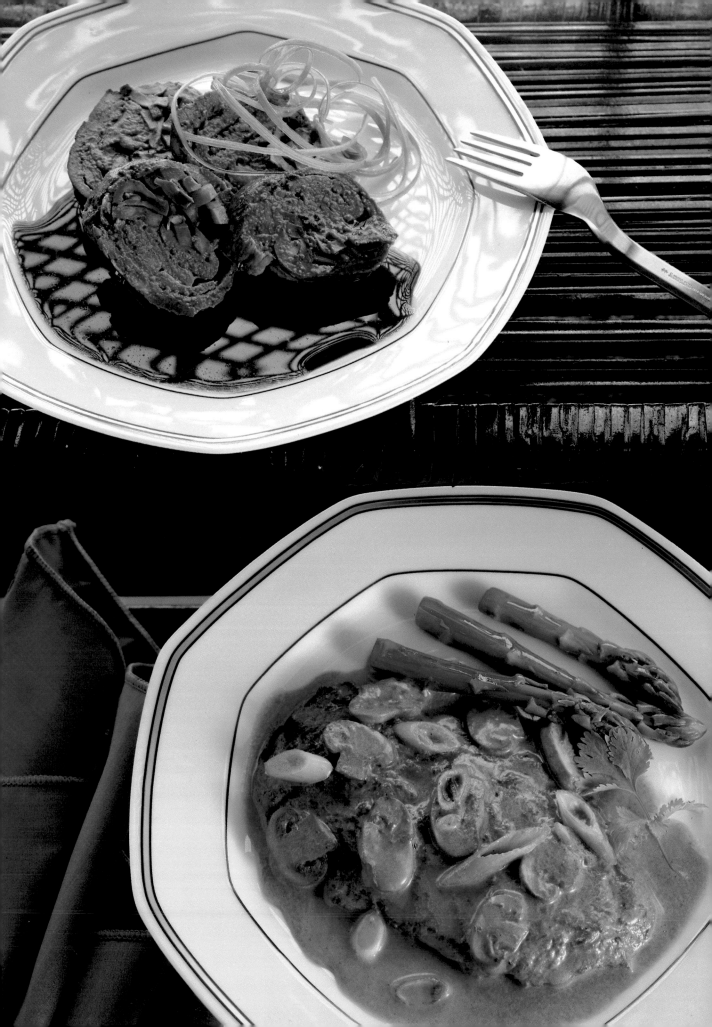

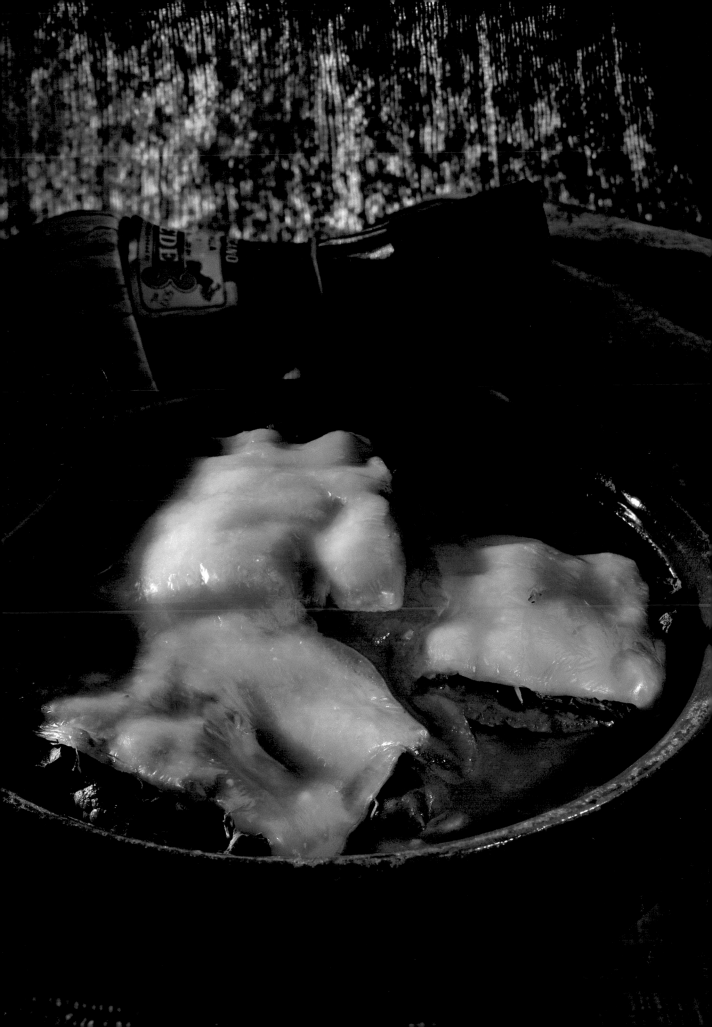

CHEESE-TOPPED VEAL WITH SPINACH

We used sliced mozzarella cheese, which is available in 250g packets. There are 6 slices in each packet. Cook dish as close to serving time as possible. This recipe is not suitable to freeze or microwave.

5 spinach (silver beet) leaves (100g)
1 tablespoon water
4 x 100g veal steaks
2 slices mozzarella cheese, halved
TOMATO SAUCE
1 teaspoon butter
1 clove garlic, crushed
310g can Tomato Supreme
¼ cup dry white wine
¼ cup water

Remove white stalks from spinach, roll leaves up tightly, shred finely. Place spinach in saucepan with water, cover, cook 5 minutes or until spinach is wilted, drain, press as much liquid as possible from the spinach.

Pound veal out thinly. Heat a large non-stick frying pan, add veal in a single layer, cook until tender. Top each piece of veal with spinach, then with a slice of mozzarella. Pour tomato sauce around the veal (do not cover cheese). Cover pan, simmer gently 10 minutes or until the cheese is melted.

Tomato Sauce: Heat butter in a saucepan, add garlic, then remaining ingredients. Bring to the boil, reduce heat, simmer, uncovered, for 5 minutes or until reduced by half.

Serves 4.

 Approximately 975 kilojoules (233 calories) per serve.

SWEET AND SPICY VEAL

This recipe is unsuitable to freeze or microwave.

2 tablespoons light soya sauce
2 tablespoons tomato sauce
2 teaspoons satay sauce
1 tablespoon dry sherry
2 teaspoons honey
1 clove garlic, crushed
2 teaspoons grated fresh ginger
250g veal steak
1 medium onion (120g), quartered
1 medium red pepper (150g), chopped
200g baby squash, quartered
200g snow peas

Combine sauces, sherry, honey, garlic and ginger in bowl. Cut veal into thin strips, add to sauce mixture, cover and refrigerate several hours or overnight. Remove veal strips from marinade and reserve marinade.

Heat a non-stick frying pan, add veal, stir constantly over heat until veal is tender, remove veal from pan.

Add vegetables to pan, stir constantly over heat until onion is just tender. Return veal and reserved marinade to pan, stir constantly until heated through.

Serves 4.

Approximately 660 kilojoules (158 calories) per serve.

VEAL IN HERB AND LEMON SAUCE

This recipe is unsuitable to freeze or microwave.

4 x 100g veal steaks
½ cup lemon juice
1 small chicken stock cube, crumbled
1 tablespoon honey
2 tablespoons brown sugar
1 teaspoon grated fresh ginger
2 cups water
1 tablespoon cornflour
1 tablespoon water, extra
1 tablespoon chopped fresh parsley
1 teaspoon chopped fresh chives
¼ teaspoon dried thyme leaves

Heat a non-stick frying pan, add veal, cook until tender, remove from pan. Add lemon juice, stock cube, honey, sugar, ginger and water to pan, bring to the boil, reduce heat, simmer, uncovered, 10 minutes. Stir in blended cornflour and extra water, stir constantly over heat until mixture boils and thickens. Add herbs to sauce, return veal to pan, cook until heated through.

Serves 4.

Approximately 660 kilojoules (158 calories) per serve.

BELOW: Left: Sweet and Spicy Veal; right: Veal in Herb and Lemon Sauce. LEFT: Cheese-Topped Veal with Spinach

Dishes & pot rack: Accoutrement

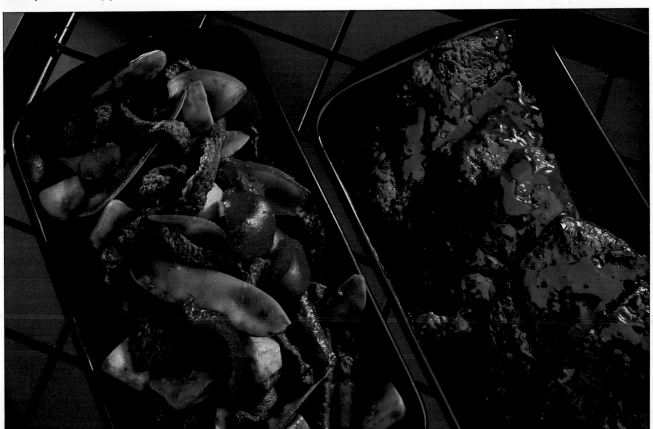

SALADS

Main course salads are a delightful way to combine many ingredients. They are nourishing and low in kilojoules. A tasty dressing, hot or cold, is always added and the salad is tossed gently in the dressing before serving. Salads should be prepared as close to serving time as possible but dressings can be prepared a day or two in advance. Salad vegetables are not suitable to freeze.

China & basket: Corso di Fiori; basket: The Australian East India Co.

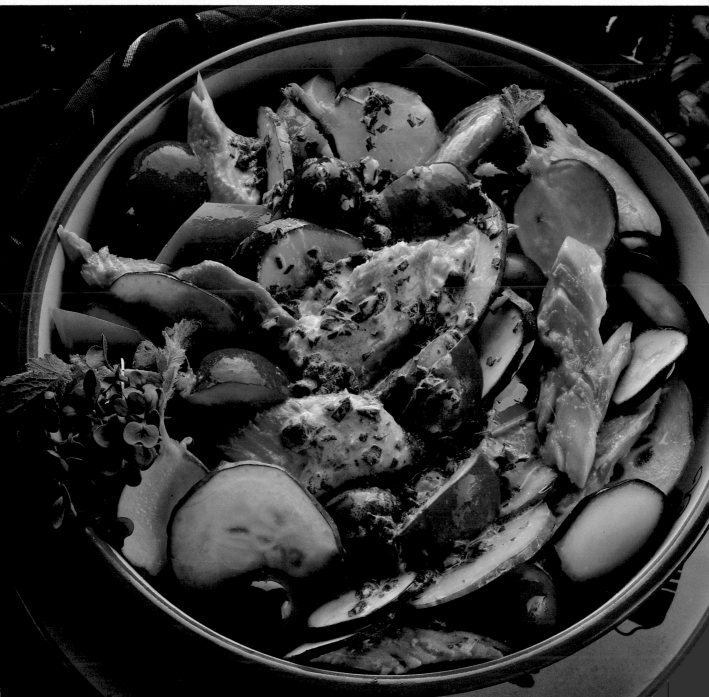

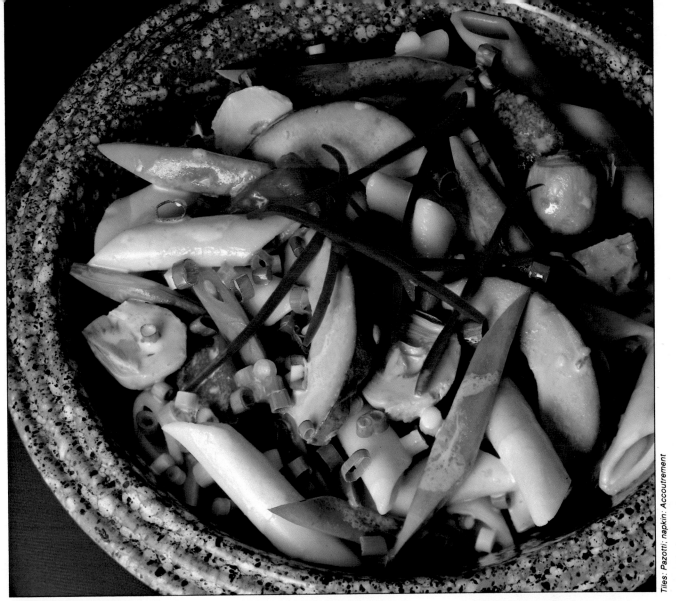

TROUT AND GARDEN VEGETABLE SALAD

Cooked fresh trout can be substituted for smoked trout, if preferred.

375g smoked trout
¼ cup lemon juice
1 medium green pepper (150g), sliced
4 small zucchini (400g), sliced
1 medium long green cucumber (280g), sliced
250g punnet cherry tomatoes
6 small radishes (120g), halved
DRESSING
2 tablespoons lemon juice
2 teaspoons oil
1 clove garlic, crushed
1 tablespoon cream
1 tablespoon chopped fresh basil
Remove skin and bones from trout, discard. Flake trout into large pieces. Combine trout, lemon juice, pepper, zucchini, cucumber, tomatoes and radishes in bowl. Add dressing just before serving.
Dressing: Combine all ingredients in screw-top jar, shake well.
Serves 4.

Approximately 695 kilojoules (166 calories) per serve.

PASTA AND AVOCADO SALAD WITH CREAMY DRESSING

1 cup penne pasta (80g)
250g green beans
3 medium tomatoes (300g)
4 canned artichokes (180g), drained, halved
1 medium avocado (200g), sliced
4 green shallots, chopped
CREAMY DRESSING
¼ cup No Oil Italian dressing
1 tablespoon low oil mayonnaise
Add pasta to saucepan of boiling water, boil, uncovered, for about 10 minutes or until just tender; drain. Top and tail beans, cut into pieces, boil, steam or microwave beans until tender; drain, rinse under cold water. Peel tomatoes, cut into wedges.

Combine pasta, beans, tomatoes, artichokes, avocado and shallots in bowl. Add dressing before serving.
Creamy Dressing: Combine dressing and mayonnaise in a small bowl, stir until smooth.
Serves 4.

Approximately 785 kilojoules (187 calories) per serve.

SEAFOOD SALAD WITH LIME AND DILL DRESSING

2 small squid hoods (250g), sliced
500g cooked king prawns, shelled
250g mussel meat, chopped
1 medium long green cucumber, (280g), sliced
4 green shallots, sliced
LIME AND DILL DRESSING
2 tablespoons lime juice
2 teaspoons oil
1 tablespoon chopped fresh dill
Drop squid into saucepan of boiling water, return to the boil, drain immediately and rinse under cold water. Combine squid, prawns, mussels, cucumber and shallots in bowl. Toss lightly in dressing just before serving.
Lime and Dill Dressing: Combine lime juice, oil and dill in a screw-top jar, shake well.
Serves 4.

Approximately 770 kilojoules (184 calories) per serve.

ABOVE: Pasta and Avocado Salad with Creamy Dressing. LEFT: Trout and Garden Vegetable Salad

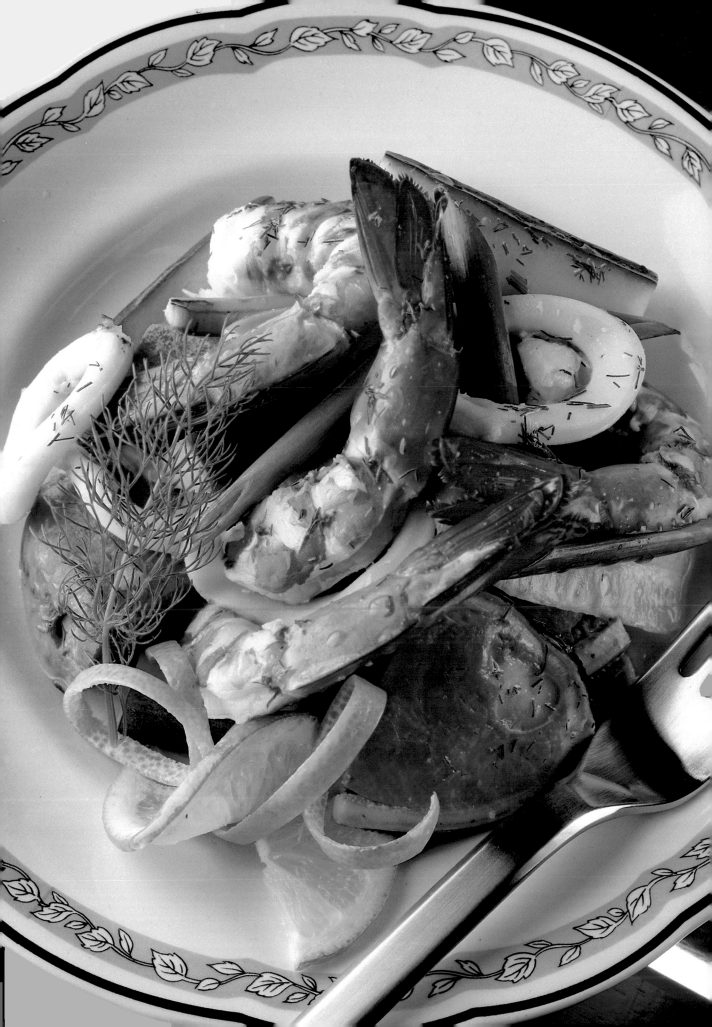

CHEESE SALAD WITH LEMON BASIL DRESSING

Use tasty cheese, if preferred.

4 medium potatoes (400g)
1 medium carrot (120g)
1 small cucumber (200g)
125g Jarlsberg cheese
8 small radishes (160g), sliced
1 bunch endive (8 leaves) (250g)
LEMON BASIL DRESSING
¼ cup lemon juice
1 tablespoon oil
½ teaspoon dried basil leaves
2 cloves garlic, crushed

Quarter potatoes, boil, steam or microwave until tender; drain, cool. Cut carrot into thin strips. Cut cucumber in half lengthways, scoop out seeds, slice cucumber thinly. Slice cheese thinly, cut into strips.

Combine potatoes, carrot, cucumber, cheese and radishes in a bowl lined with endive. Add dressing just before serving, toss lightly.

Lemon Basil Dressing: Combine ingredients in screw-top jar; shake well.

Serves 4.

Approximately 1020 kilojoules (244 calories) per serve.

LEFT: Seafood Salad with Lime and Dill Dressing. RIGHT: Cheese Salad with Lemon Basil Dressing. BELOW: Smoked Cod and Brown Rice Salad

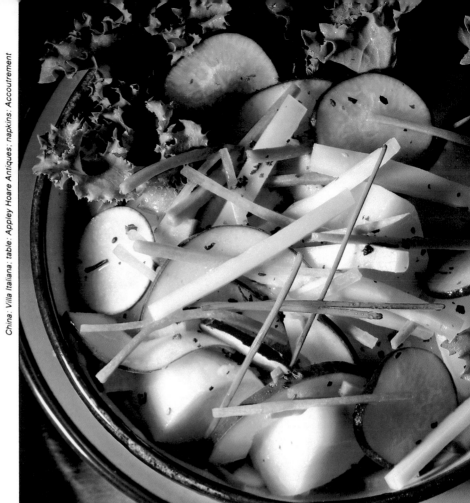

China: Villa Italiana: table: Appley Hoare Antiques; napkins: Accoutrement

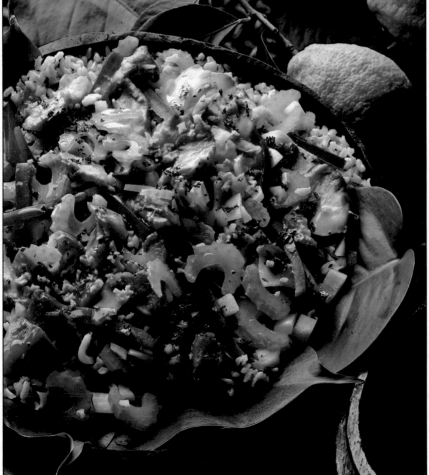

Bowl & basket: Corso di Fiori

SMOKED COD AND BROWN RICE SALAD

1¼ cups brown rice (250g)
250g smoked cod
1 small stick celery (60g), sliced
1 small red pepper (100g), sliced
1 small onion (80g), finely chopped
DRESSING
2 tablespoons chopped fresh parsley
1 teaspoon grated fresh ginger
1 teaspoon French mustard
½ cup No Oil French dressing

Add rice gradually to a large saucepan of boiling water, boil rapidly, uncovered, for 30 minutes, or until tender; drain, cool.

Place cod in frying pan, cover with cold water, bring to the boil, remove from heat; drain, cool. Break cod into flakes, combine in bowl with rice, celery, pepper and onion. Pour dressing over salad just before serving.

Dressing: Combine parsley, ginger, mustard and dressing in screw-top jar, shake well.

Serves 4.

Approximately 1200 kilojoules (287 calories) per serve.

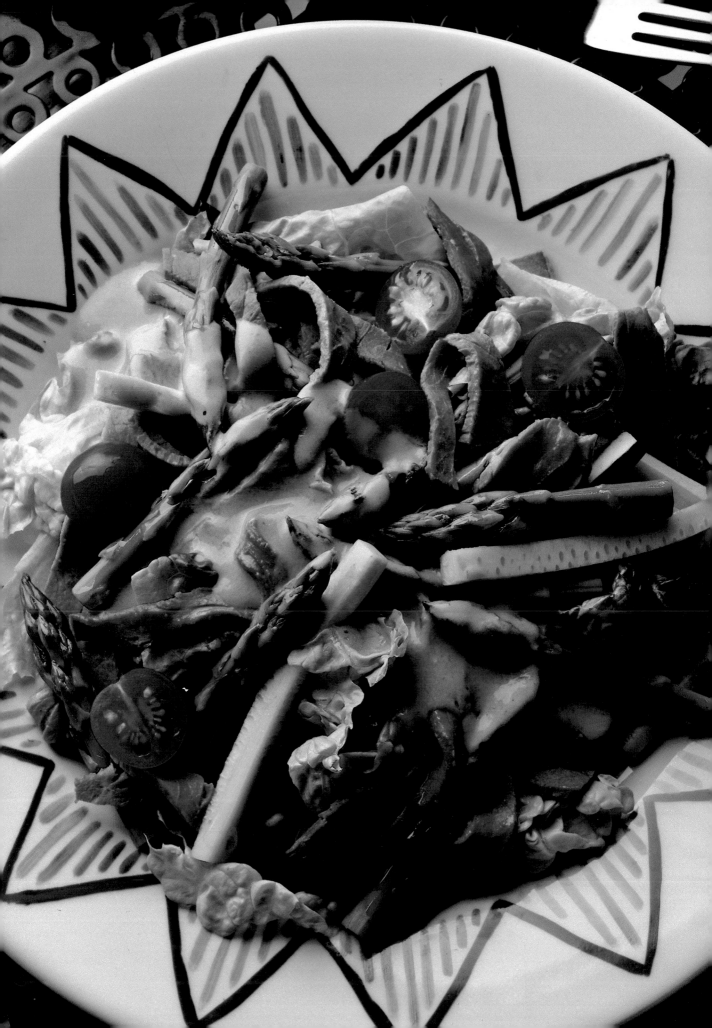

SWEET AND SOUR FISH

We used bream fillets for this recipe. You will need to cook two-thirds cup of rice for this recipe; it is not suitable to freeze.

4 x 125g white fish fillets
1 medium carrot (120g)
1 small red pepper (100g)
1 medium onion (120g)
2 teaspoons oil
½ small cucumber (100g), chopped
1 large stick celery (100g), thinly sliced
2 teaspoons cornflour
¾ cup water
2 tablespoons tomato sauce
1 teaspoon light soya sauce
1 tablespoon brown sugar
1 tablespoon brown vinegar
2 cups cooked rice

Steam, poach or microwave fish until tender. Cut carrot and pepper into thin strips. Cut onion into quarters.

Heat oil in frying pan, add vegetables, stir constantly over heat until onion is soft. Blend cornflour with water, stir in sauces, sugar and vinegar, add to pan, stir constantly over heat until mixture boils and thickens. Place fish over rice, top with sauce.

Serves 4.

Approximately 1105 kilojoules (264 calories) per serve.

STIR-FRIED GINGER SEAFOOD

We used bream fillets for this recipe. This dish can be frozen for up to a month; it is not suitable to microwave.

500g white fish fillets
6 spinach (silver beet) leaves (120g)
375g cooked medium prawns
2 teaspoons oil
1 tablespoon chopped fresh ginger
SAUCE
2 teaspoons cornflour
¼ cup water
2 teaspoons light soya sauce
½ small chicken stock cube, crumbled

Cut fish into 2cm pieces. Remove white stalks from centre of spinach, cut leaves into 4cm pieces. Shell prawns, remove dark vein.

Drop spinach into a saucepan of boiling water, drain immediately, place onto serving plates; keep warm. Heat oil in a wok or frying pan, add ginger, fish and prawns; stir-fry over high heat until fish is just tender. Add sauce, stir constantly until mixture boils and thickens, spoon over spinach.

Sauce: Blend cornflour in bowl with water, add soya sauce and stock cube.

Serves 4.

Approximately 760 kilojoules (182 calories) per serve.

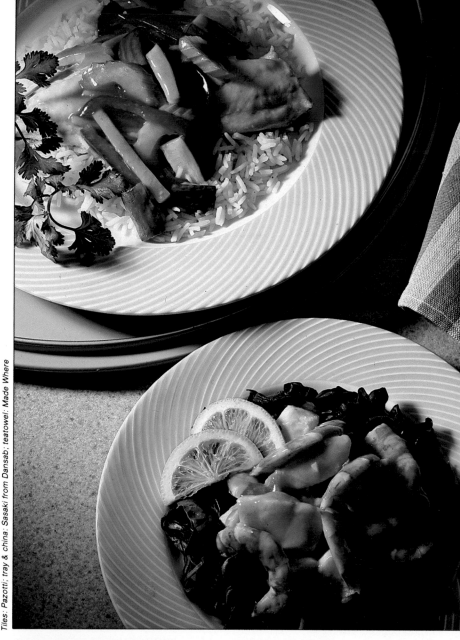

Tiles: Pazotti; tray & china: Sasaki from Dansab; teatowel: Made Where

CORIANDER FISH KEBABS

We used ling fish for this recipe. If using wooden skewers, soak them in cold water overnight to help prevent burning during cooking. This recipe is not suitable to freeze or microwave.

500g white fish fillets
MARINADE
1 tablespoon oil
1 clove garlic, crushed
1 small fresh red chilli, finely chopped
½ teaspoon sugar
2 tablespoons chopped fresh coriander
2 teaspoons grated fresh ginger
1 teaspoon paprika
½ teaspoon ground cumin
2 teaspoons grated lemon rind
⅓ cup lemon juice
YOGHURT SAUCE
1 small cucumber (200g), peeled
salt
½ cup low-fat plain yoghurt
1 tablespoon chopped fresh coriander

Cut fish into large chunks, place in bowl, add marinade, mix well, cover, refrigerate 4 hours or overnight. Thread fish onto skewers, barbecue or grill gently, basting with marinade until fish is tender. Serve with sauce.

Marinade: Combine all ingredients in bowl, mix well.

Yoghurt Sauce: Remove seeds from cucumber, chop cucumber roughly, place in strainer, sprinkle with salt. Stand cucumber 15 minutes, rinse under cold water, pat dry. Blend or process yoghurt, cucumber and coriander until smooth.

Serves 4.

Approximately 780 kilojoules (186 calories) per serve.

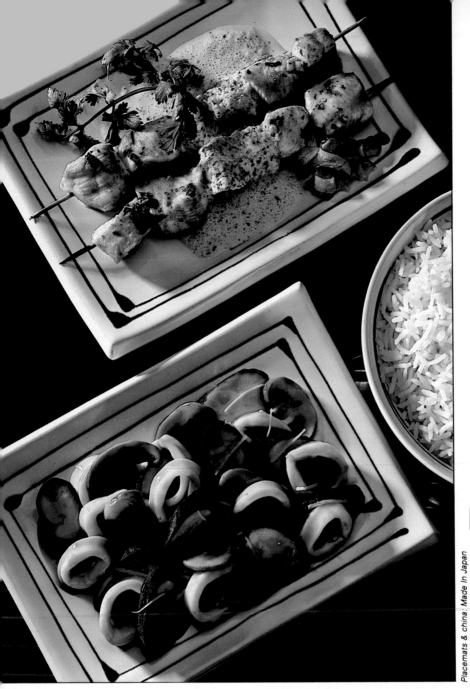

SMOKED COD AND CORN WITH BROWN RICE

We used fresh corn in this recipe, but canned, drained, whole kernel corn can be used, if preferred. You will need to cook two-thirds cup of brown rice. This dish is not suitable to freeze.

400g smoked cod
¾ cup fresh corn kernels
½ cup water
1 large carrot (200g), grated
2 cups cooked brown rice
230g can water chestnuts, drained,
chopped
1 tablespoon light soya sauce
6 green shallots, chopped
½ cup low-fat plain yoghurt

Place cod in frying pan, add enough water to cover cod, bring to the boil, reduce heat, simmer, uncovered, for about 10 minutes (or microwave on HIGH for about 3 minutes). Drain cod, discard skin and bones and flake cod with fork.

Boil, steam or microwave corn until tender, drain. Heat water in a large frying pan, add carrot, cook 1 minute, stir in rice, corn, water chestnuts and soya sauce, stir until heated through. Stir in cod, shallots and yoghurt, reheat gently, stirring constantly (or microwave on HIGH for about 5 minutes).

Serves 4.

Approximately 950 kilojoules (227 calories) per serve.

Placemats & china: Made in Japan

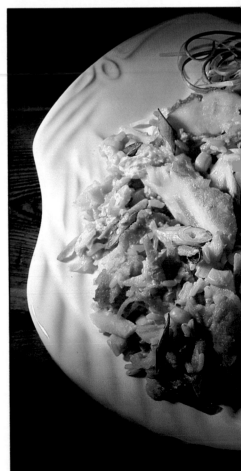

STIR-FRIED SQUID IN LEMON GINGER SAUCE

This recipe is not suitable to freeze or microwave.

750g squid
2cm piece fresh ginger, peeled
2 teaspoons oil
3 medium zucchini (450g), sliced
250g mushrooms, sliced
SAUCE
2 teaspoons cornflour
2 teaspoons sugar
2 tablespoons lemon juice
1 small chicken stock cube, crumbled
1 tablespoon light soya sauce
½ cup water

ABOVE: Top: Coriander Fish Kebabs; bottom: Stir-Fried Squid in Lemon Ginger Sauce. RIGHT: Smoked Cod and Corn with Brown Rice

Hold squid with one hand, hold head and pull gently with other hand. Head and inside of body of squid will come away in a complete piece. Remove bone which will be found at open end of squid; it looks like a long piece of plastic. Clean squid under cold water, then rub off outer skin. Cut squid evenly into rings.

Cut ginger into wafer-thin slices, then cut into fine shreds. Drop squid into saucepan of boiling water, boil 10 seconds, drain immediately. Heat oil in wok or frying pan, add zucchini, stir-fry 2 minutes, add ginger, squid and mushrooms, stir-fry 2 minutes. Add sauce; stir constantly until mixture boils and thickens.

Sauce: Blend cornflour and sugar in small bowl with lemon juice, stir in remaining ingredients.

Serves 4.

Approximately 840 kilojoules (200 calories) per serve.

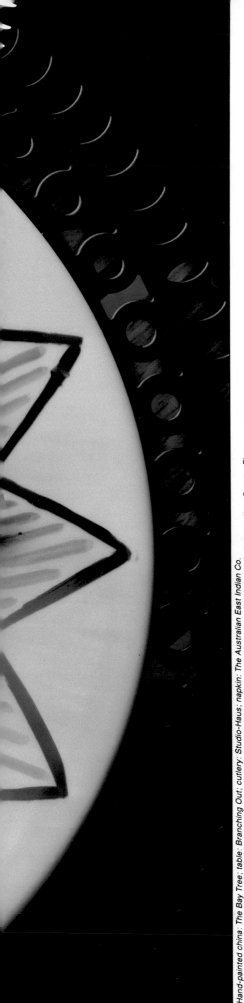

RARE ROAST BEEF AND ASPARAGUS SALAD

250g beef eye fillet in one piece
250g fresh asparagus
2 small zucchini (200g), sliced
250g punnet cherry tomatoes, halved
1 mignonette lettuce
DRESSING
¼ cup low-fat plain yoghurt
1½ tablespoons tomato sauce
½ teaspoon Worcestershire sauce

Tie the beef with string to hold in shape during cooking, place in baking dish, bake in hot oven for 10 minutes, reduce heat to moderate and bake further 20 minutes, or until cooked as desired. Cool beef, cut in strips.

Boil, steam or microwave asparagus until just tender, place into bowl of iced water; drain, cut asparagus in half. Combine beef, asparagus, zucchini, tomatoes and lettuce in bowl. Pour dressing over salad before serving.

Dressing: Combine yoghurt and sauces in bowl.

Serves 4.

Approximately 560 kilojoules (133 calories) per serve.

HOT SPINACH BACON SALAD

2 bacon rashers (80g), chopped
40 English spinach leaves
3 hard-boiled eggs, chopped
2 green shallots, sliced
250g punnet cherry tomatoes
DRESSING
⅓ cup No Oil French dressing
1 teaspoon oil

Cook bacon in small frying pan until crisp; drain on absorbent paper. Tear spinach into bite-sized pieces, place in serving bowl, add eggs, shallots, tomatoes and bacon. Pour dressing over salad just before serving.

Dressing: Combine dressing and oil in saucepan, bring to the boil, remove from heat.

Serves 4.

Approximately 750 kilojoules (180 calories) per serve.

BELOW: Hot Spinach Bacon Salad. LEFT: Rare Roast Beef and Asparagus Salad

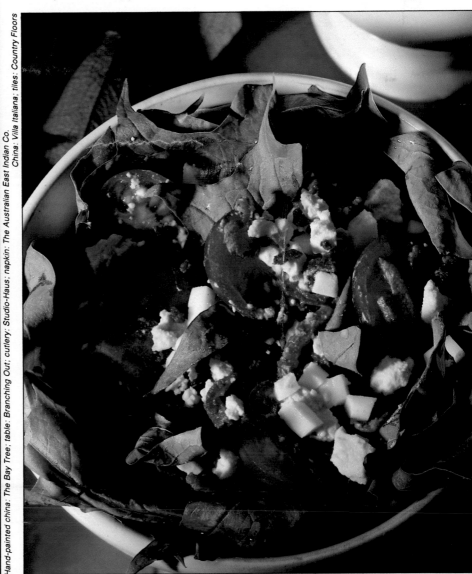

Hand-painted china: The Bay Tree; table: Branching Out; cutlery: Studio-Haus; napkin: The Australian East Indian Co. China: Villa Italiana; tiles: Country Floors

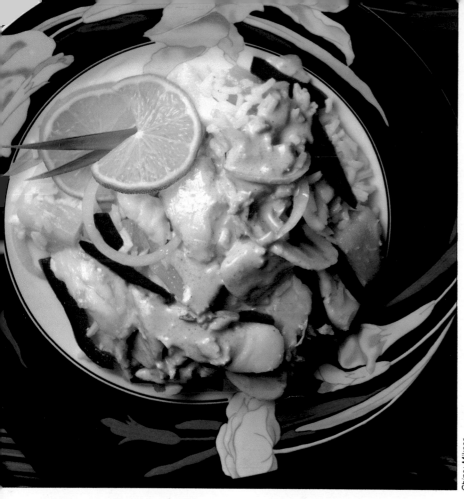

China: Mikasa

TROPICAL FISH SALAD WITH COCONUT CREAM DRESSING

We used ling fillets in this dish. You will need to cook quarter cup of rice first.

500g white fish fillets
¾ cup cooked rice
½ cup drained unsweetened pineapple pieces
1 small onion (80g), thinly sliced
1 medium red pepper (150g), thinly sliced
1 small banana (100g), sliced
1 tablespoon lemon juice
COCONUT CREAM DRESSING
⅓ cup coconut cream
2 tablespoons low oil mayonnaise
1 tablespoon lemon juice
2 teaspoons sugar
1 teaspoon grated fresh ginger
1 teaspoon curry powder

Boil, steam or microwave fish until tender; drain. Remove bones and skin from fish, break into chunks, cool to room temperature. Combine fish with remaining ingredients, refrigerate several hours. Pour dressing over salad just before serving.

Coconut Cream Dressing: Combine all ingredients in bowl, mix well.

Serves 4.

Approximately 1040 kilojoules (248 calories) per serve.

ABOVE: Tropical Fish Salad with Coconut Cream Dressing. RIGHT: Chicken and Pasta Salad

CHICKEN AND PASTA SALAD

115g chicken breast fillet
220g fettucine
2 teaspoons sesame seeds
100g snow peas
125g broccoli
1 medium green pepper (150g), sliced
6 green shallots, chopped
DRESSING
¼ cup lemon juice
1 tablespoon French mustard
1 tablespoon chopped fresh parsley
2 teaspoons grated fresh ginger
¼ cup water

Poach, steam or microwave chicken until tender; drain, cool, slice finely.

Add fettucine to large saucepan of boiling water, boil rapidly, uncovered, for about 10 minutes, or until just tender; drain. Rinse fettucine under cold water; drain.

Toast sesame seeds on oven tray in moderate oven or frying pan; cool.

Drop snow peas and broccoli into saucepan of boiling water, return to boil, drain, place into bowl of iced water; drain.

Place fettucine onto serving plate, top with snow peas, broccoli, pepper, shallots and chicken, sprinkle with sesame seeds. Add dressing just before serving.

Dressing: Combine all ingredients in a screw-top jar; shake well.

Serves 4.

Approximately 1230 kilojoules (294 calories) per serve.

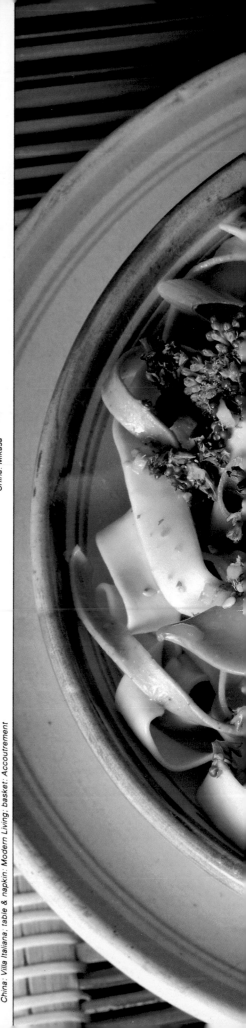

China: Villa Italiana; table & napkin: Modern Living; basket: Accoutrement

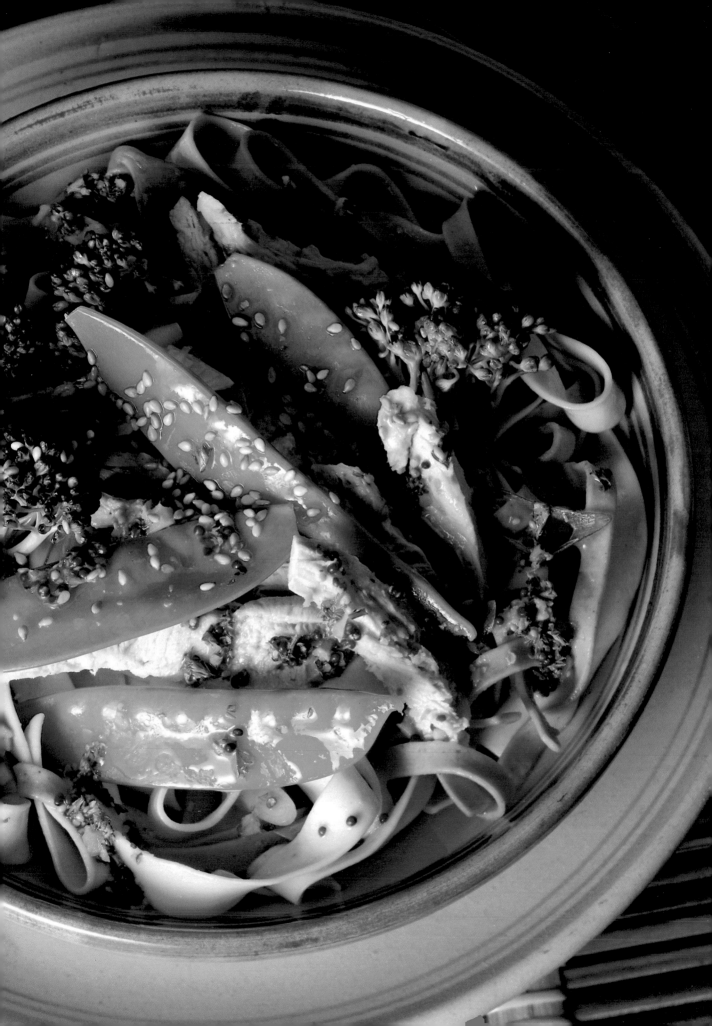

TUNA SALAD WITH LEMON PEPPER DRESSING

You will need to cook 50g pasta for this recipe. This recipe is not suitable to freeze.

100g green beans
12 radishes (240g), quartered
1 medium onion (120g), thinly sliced
2 x 185g cans tuna in brine, drained
1¼ cups cooked pasta
LEMON PEPPER DRESSING
½ cup low oil mayonnaise
2 teaspoons canned green
    peppercorns, drained, crushed
2 teaspoons lemon juice
1 teaspoon grated lemon rind
½ teaspoon sugar

Top and tail beans and cut into 2cm lengths. Boil, steam or microwave beans until just tender; drain. Combine beans with the remaining ingredients in a bowl. Add dressing to salad just before serving.

Lemon Pepper Dressing: Combine ingredients in small bowl; mix well.

Serves 4.

Approximately 830 kilojoules (198 calories) per serve.

BELOW: Top: Tuna Salad with Lemon Pepper Dressing; bottom: Chick Pea and Mint Salad. RIGHT: Left: Bean and Barley Salad with Mint Dressing; right: Vitality Tofu Salad

CHICK PEA AND MINT SALAD

You will need to soak 325g dried chick peas in cold water overnight before cooking. Chick peas can be prepared up to 3 days ahead, store, covered, in refrigerator. This recipe is not suitable to freeze or microwave.

4 cups soaked chick peas
    (garbanzos)
1 green shallot, chopped
1 medium long green cucumber
    (280g), chopped
1 medium red pepper (150g),
    chopped
1 medium stick celery (80g),
    chopped
1 medium carrot (120g), chopped
1 tablespoon chopped fresh mint
2 teaspoons chopped fresh
    coriander
DRESSING
2 teaspoons light soya sauce
1 tablespoon lemon juice
2 tablespoons orange juice
1 small fresh red chilli, chopped
1 clove garlic, crushed

Boil chick peas in a large saucepan of water for about 1 hour, or until tender; drain, cool.

Combine chick peas, shallot, cucumber, pepper, celery, carrot, mint and coriander in a bowl. Add dressing just before serving.

Dressing: Combine all ingredients in a small bowl; mix well.

Serves 4.

Approximately 1225 kilojoules (293 calories) per serve.

BEAN AND BARLEY SALAD WITH MINT DRESSING

Use 250g frozen broad beans if fresh are unavailable. This recipe is unsuitable to freeze.

¾ cup barley (150g)
500g broad beans, shelled
310g can red kidney beans, rinsed,
    drained
2 medium sticks celery (160g), sliced
1 small red pepper (100g), sliced
MINT DRESSING
60g packaged cream cheese,
    softened
⅓ cup mint leaves, firmly packed
2 tablespoons lemon juice
1 tablespoon skim milk
1 clove garlic, crushed

Cook barley in boiling water for about 15 minutes, or until tender; drain. Boil, steam or microwave broad beans until tender; drain, rinse under cold water, drain. Combine barley, broad beans, kidney beans, celery and pepper in a bowl; add dressing just before serving.

Mint Dressing: Blend or process all ingredients until smooth.

Serves 4.

Approximately 1255 kilojoules (300 calories) per serve.

VITALITY TOFU SALAD

Tofu, or packaged soya bean curd, is available at health food stores, Chinese specialty shops and some supermarkets. Recipe unsuitable to freeze or microwave.

375g solid tofu, cubed
200g oyster (abalone) mushrooms
1 cup alfalfa sprouts (40g)
1 cup bean sprouts (60g)
440g can whole baby carrots,
    drained
1 medium red pepper (150g),
    chopped
2 medium zucchini (300g) sliced
425g can baby corn, drained
CITRUS DRESSING
2 teaspoons oil
¼ teaspoon sesame oil
1 tablespoon lemon juice
1 tablespoon lime juice
¼ teaspoon dark soya sauce
2 teaspoons brown sugar

Combine tofu, mushrooms, sprouts, halved carrots, pepper, zucchini and corn in bowl, add the dressing just before serving.

Citrus Dressing: Combine all ingredients in screw-top jar, shake well.

Serves 4.

Approximately 1015 kilojoules (243 calories) per serve.

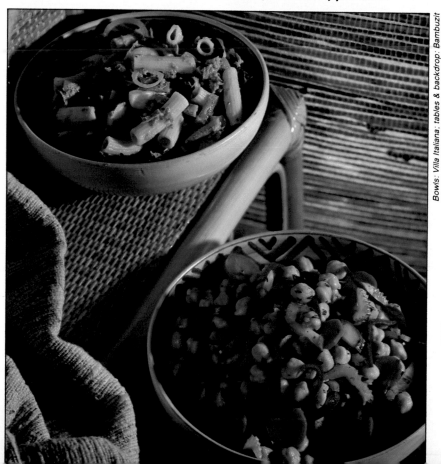

Bowls: Villa Italiana; tables & backdrop: Bambuzit

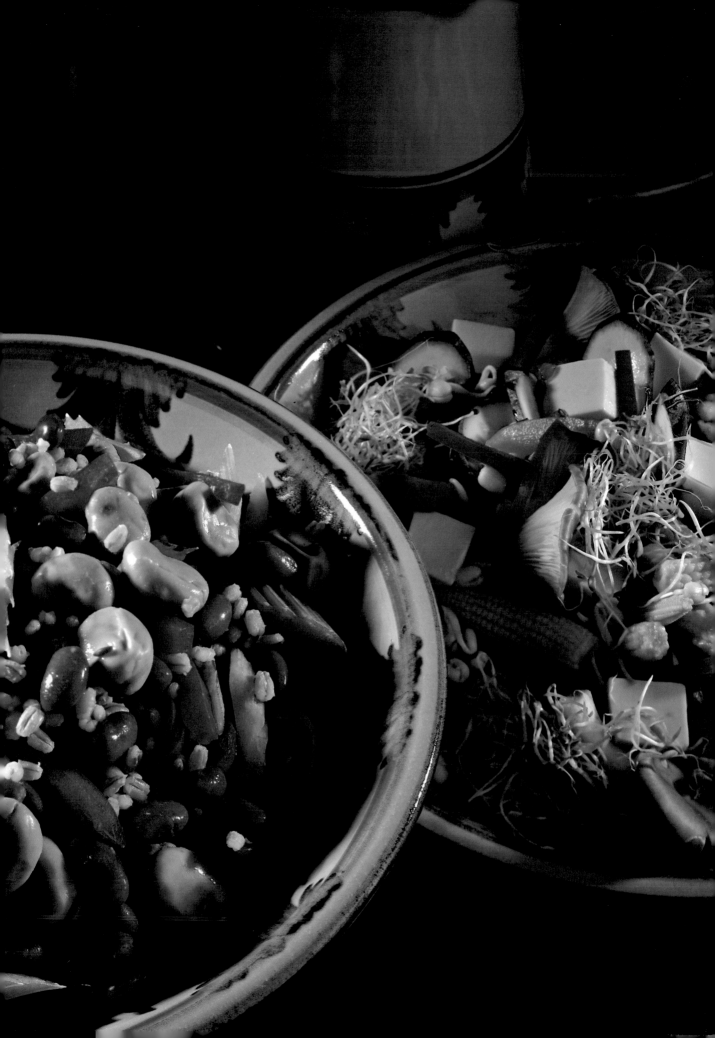

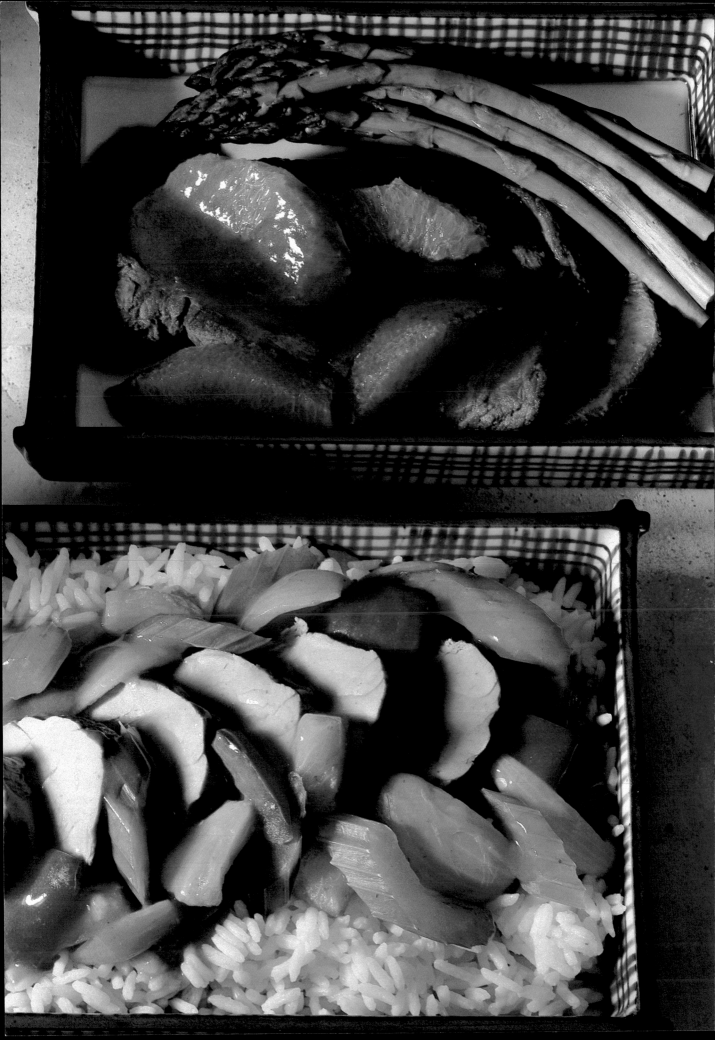

PORK

Pork is recognised as a white meat which is low in fat; any small amount of visible fat should be trimmed off before cooking. Most of the recipes in this section use pork fillet because there is no bone or fat and it is quick and easy to cook. However, pork steaks or any suitable cut can be used, although the kilojoule count will be slightly higher.

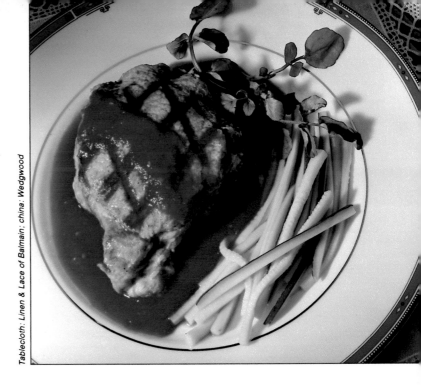

Tablecloth: Linen & Lace of Balmain; china: Wedgwood

FRUITY GLAZED PORK

This recipe is not suitable to freeze or microwave.

1 large orange (220g)
½ cup apricot nectar
2 tablespoons orange juice
2 teaspoons brown sugar
1 small chicken stock cube, crumbled
2 teaspoons Worcestershire sauce
4 x 100g pork steaks
1 teaspoon cornflour
1 tablespoon water

Peel orange thickly, remove as much white pith as possible. Cut orange into segments, cutting between membranes, discard seeds and fibrous material in centre. Combine orange segments, apricot nectar, orange juice, sugar, stock cube and Worcestershire sauce in bowl, add steaks, cover, refrigerate several hours or overnight. Next day, drain steaks, reserve marinade, reserve orange segments.

Place steaks in heated frying pan, cook on both sides until tender. Remove steaks from pan.

Place reserved marinade in pan, stir in blended cornflour and water, stir constantly over heat until mixture boils and thickens. Return steaks and orange segments to pan and reheat.
Serves 4.

Approximately 700 kilojoules (167 calories) per serve.

SWEET AND SOUR PORK

Recipe can be frozen for up to 2 months. You will need to cook two-thirds cup of rice for this recipe.

440g can unsweetened pineapple pieces
1 tablespoon brown vinegar
1 teaspoon light soya sauce
1½ tablespoons tomato sauce
400g pork fillets
4 small onions (320g), quartered
1 medium red pepper (150g), chopped
2 medium sticks celery (160g), sliced
2 teaspoons cornflour
1 tablespoon water
2 cups cooked rice

Combine undrained pineapple, vinegar and sauces in an oven bag with pork, onions, pepper and celery, seal bag as directed on packet. Place in baking dish, bake in moderate oven for about 45 minutes, or until pork and vegetables are tender (or microwave on HIGH for about 15 minutes).

Cut bag open, remove pork and vegetables, pour juices into baking dish, bring to the boil, boil rapidly until reduced by about one-third. Stir in blended cornflour and water, stir constantly over heat until sauce boils and thickens. Serve sliced pork and vegetables over rice, top with sauce.
Serves 4.

Approximately 1255 kilojoules (300 calories) per serve.

BUTTERFLY PORK POCKETS WITH PIMIENTO SAUCE

This recipe is not suitable to freeze or microwave.

4 x 175g pork butterfly steaks
4 large spinach (silver beet) leaves (100g)
⅓ cup ricotta cheese (75g)
4 green shallots, chopped
1 clove garlic, crushed
15g butter
PIMIENTO SAUCE
2 whole canned pimientos (120g), drained, chopped
1 medium tomato (100g), peeled, chopped
1 medium onion (120g), chopped
1 cup water
1 tablespoon tomato paste

Open steaks out flat. Boil, steam or microwave spinach until just tender, drain, squeeze out excess liquid, chop spinach roughly. Combine spinach, cheese, shallots and garlic in bowl; mix well. Spread evenly over steaks. Fold steaks over, secure with toothpicks.

Heat butter in frying pan, add steaks, fry on both sides until browned. Place steaks in a single layer in an ovenproof dish, bake, uncovered, in moderate oven for about 20 minutes, or until tender. Serve with sauce.
Pimiento Sauce: Combine pimientos, tomato, onion, water and tomato paste in a saucepan, bring to the boil, cover, reduce heat, simmer for 10 minutes (or microwave on HIGH about 10 minutes). Blend or process until smooth, strain, reheat sauce before serving.
Serves 4.

Approximately 1185 kilojoules (283 calories) per serve.

LEFT: Top: Fruity Glazed Pork; bottom: Sweet and Sour Pork. ABOVE: Butterfly Pork Pockets with Pimiento Sauce

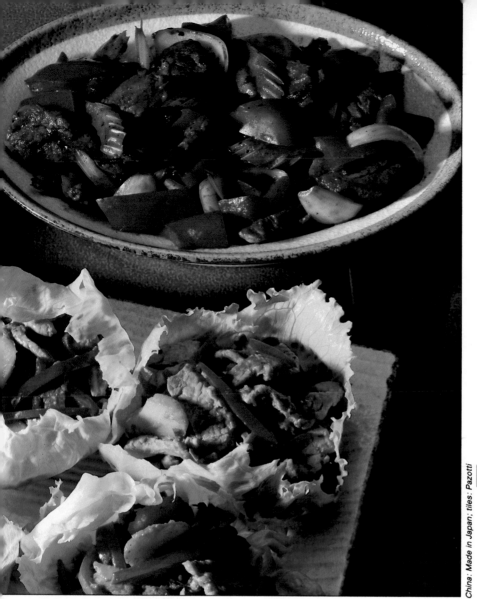

China: Made in Japan; tiles: Pazotti

BARBECUED PORK STIR-FRY

This recipe is not suitable to freeze or microwave.

2 tablespoons tomato sauce
2 teaspoons light soya sauce
1 tablespoon white vinegar
1 tablespoon dry sherry
1 tablespoon brown sugar
1 teaspoon grated fresh ginger
1 clove garlic, crushed
300g pork fillets, thinly sliced
2 teaspoons oil
1 medium onion (120g), chopped
1 stick celery (100g), sliced
1 medium red pepper, chopped (150g)
2 teaspoons cornflour
1 cup water

Combine sauces, vinegar, sherry, sugar, ginger and garlic in bowl, add pork, cover, refrigerate 1 hour.

Remove pork from marinade, drain well, reserve marinade. Heat oil in a frying pan or wok, add pork, stir-fry until pork is tender. Remove pork from pan, add onion, celery and pepper, stir-fry until onion is soft. Blend cornflour with water in bowl, add marinade, add to pan with pork, stir-fry until mixture boils and thickens.
Serves 4.

Approximately 675 kilojoules (161 calories) per serve.

PORK WITH APPLE SAUCE

Recipe unsuitable to freeze.

1 teaspoon curry powder
1 clove garlic, crushed
1 teaspoon French mustard
400g pork fillets
APPLE SAUCE
10 dried apple rings (25g)
1 small chicken stock cube, crumbled
¼ cup dry white wine
1 teaspoon cornflour
¾ cup water

Combine curry powder, garlic and mustard, spread evenly over pork; cover and refrigerate several hours or overnight to allow flavour to develop. Place pork in baking dish, bake in moderate oven for 15 minutes (or microwave on HIGH about 5 minutes).

Top with apple sauce, bake further 5 minutes (or microwave on HIGH for about 5 minutes) or until tender.
Apple Sauce: Combine apple rings, stock cube, wine and blended cornflour and water in a saucepan, stir constantly over heat until mixture boils and thickens, reduce heat and simmer, uncovered, 10 minutes (or microwave on HIGH for about 4 minutes).
Serves 4.

Approximately 575 kilojoules (137 calories) per serve.

CHILLI PORK STIR-FRY

This recipe will freeze for up to 2 months; it is not suitable to microwave.

400g pork fillets
1 medium red pepper (150g)
2 teaspoons oil
1 clove garlic, crushed
1 tablespoon grated fresh ginger
1 small fresh red chilli, finely chopped
¼ cup water
1 tablespoon light soya sauce
6 canned water chestnuts (50g), sliced
4 lettuce cups

Cut pork and pepper into strips. Heat oil in a wok or frying pan; add garlic, ginger, chilli and pork, stir-fry until tender, remove from pan. Add pepper, stir-fry until just tender, remove from pan. Add water and soya sauce to pan, boil until reduced by half. Return pork and pepper to pan with water chestnuts, stir-fry until heated through. Serve in lettuce cups.
Serves 4.

Approximately 660 kilojoules (157 calories) per serve.

PORK IN GINGER PLUM SAUCE

Recipe unsuitable to freeze.

400g pork fillets
2 teaspoons butter
GINGER PLUM SAUCE
1 small onion (80g), finely chopped
1 teaspoon grated fresh ginger
1 clove garlic, crushed
¼ cup water
2 canned plums (100g)
¼ cup syrup from canned plums
3 teaspoons brandy

Slice pork thinly. Heat butter in a frying pan, add pork, cook, stirring constantly, until lightly browned and tender; drain away any liquid. Serve with ginger plum sauce.
Ginger Plum Sauce: Combine onion, ginger, garlic and water in a saucepan, stir constantly over heat until onion is soft (or microwave on HIGH for about 5 minutes). Add plums, syrup and brandy, bring to the boil, reduce heat, simmer 1 minute (or microwave on HIGH for about 2 minutes). Blend or process until smooth. Reheat before serving.
Serves 4.

Approximately 665 kilojoules (158 calories) per serve.

CURRIED PORK FILLET

This recipe is not suitable to freeze or microwave.

1 tablespoon sweet mango chutney
400g pork fillets
2 teaspoons oil
1 small onion (80g), chopped
1 teaspoon curry powder
1 tablespoon sultanas
1 teaspoon cornflour
¾ cup water

Brush chutney evenly over pork. Heat oil in baking dish, add pork, cook over high heat until lightly browned all over. Bake in moderate oven for about 25 minutes, or until pork is tender, brush pork with pan drippings during cooking. Remove from dish; keep warm.

Place baking dish on top of stove over medium heat. Add onion and curry powder, cook, stirring constantly, until onion is soft, stir in sultanas. Gradually stir in blended cornflour and water, stir constantly over heat until sauce boils and thickens; serve over sliced pork.

Serves 4.

Approximately 685 kilojoules (164 calories) per serve.

BELOW: Clockwise from top: Curried Pork Fillet; Pork in Ginger Plum Sauce; Pork with Apple Sauce. OPPOSITE PAGE: Top: Barbecued Pork Stir-Fry; bottom: Chilli Pork Stir-Fry

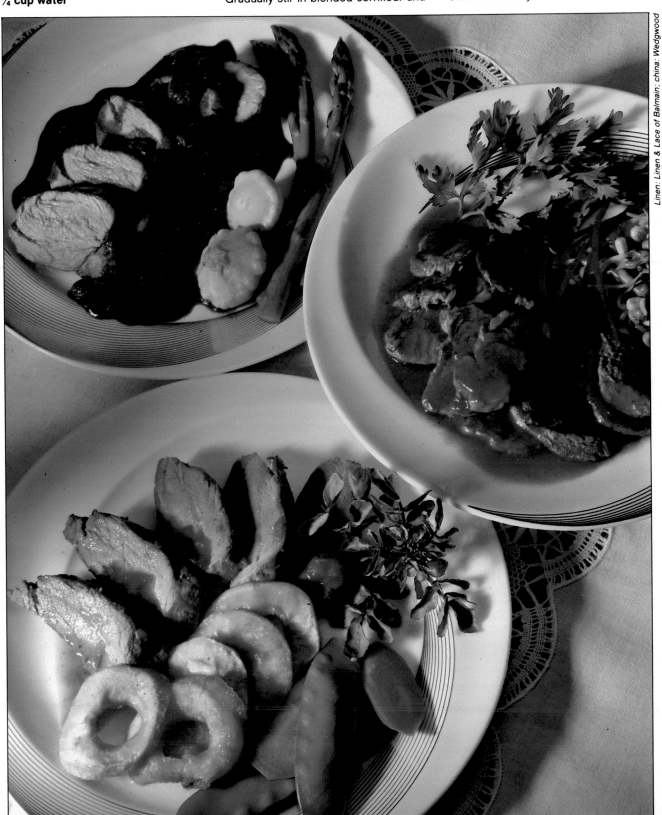

Linen: Linen & Lace of Balmain; china: Wedgwood

PORK STEAKS WITH GREEN PEPPERCORN SAUCE

This recipe is unsuitable to freeze or microwave.

2 x 200g pork butterfly steaks
1 teaspoon oil
1 teaspoon canned green peppercorns, drained, crushed
2 tablespoons dry sherry
½ cup evaporated skim milk
1 teaspoon cornflour
1 teaspoon water

Cut steaks in half. Heat oil in a frying pan, add steaks, cook until tender, remove from pan, keep warm.

Add peppercorns and sherry to pan, stir in combined milk and blended cornflour and water. Stir constantly over heat until mixture boils and thickens. Serve with steaks.

Serves 4.

Approximately 835 kilojoules (200 calories) per serve.

STIR-FRIED PORK AND VEGETABLES

Recipe unsuitable to freeze.

4 x 100g pork steaks
1 tablespoon tomato sauce
1 tablespoon light soya sauce
2 teaspoons honey
¼ teaspoon five spice powder
2 medium carrots (240g)
3 small zucchini (300g)

Cut pork into thin strips, combine in a bowl with sauces, honey and five spice powder; stand 30 minutes.

Cut carrots and zucchini into thin strips, boil, steam or microwave until just tender; drain, rinse under cold water, drain.

Heat a non-stick frying pan or wok, add pork gradually to pan, stir-fry over high heat until pork is browned and tender. Add carrot and zucchini, stir-fry over high heat until heated through.

Serves 4.

Approximately 575 kilojoules (137 calories) per serve.

PORK IN BLACK BEAN SAUCE

Bottled black bean sauce is available at Asian food stores. This recipe unsuitable to freeze or microwave.

4 x 100g pork steaks
¼ cup black bean sauce
1 teaspoon chilli sauce
1 teaspoon oil
1 small leek (150g), thinly sliced
2 teaspoons cornflour
2 tablespoons water

Cut pork into fine strips, combine in bowl with sauces, refrigerate for 2 hours or overnight.

Heat oil in wok or frying pan, add leek, stir-fry over low heat until tender. Remove from pan. Add pork to pan, stir-fry until tender, return leek to pan, stir in blended cornflour and water, stir-fry until mixture boils and thickens.

Serves 4.

Approximately 670 kilojoules (160 calories) per serve.

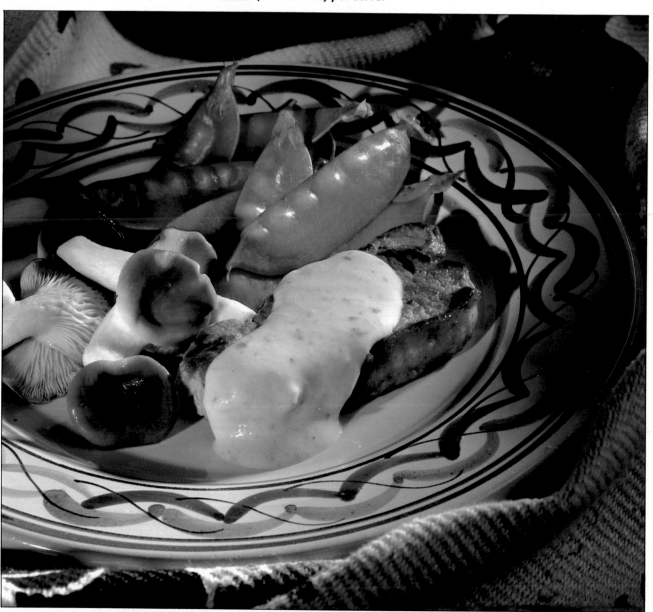

Plate: Villa Italiana; rug: Mosmania

CABBAGE PORK ROLLS

This recipe is not suitable to freeze.

250g pork steaks, chopped
230g can water chestnuts, drained
2 green shallots, chopped
1 clove garlic, crushed
2 medium sticks celery (160g),
chopped
1 medium carrot (120g), chopped
2 teaspoons oyster sauce
3 teaspoons cornflour
4 large cabbage leaves
8 fresh chives
CORIANDER SAUCE
¾ cup water
1 small chicken stock cube, crumbled
1 green shallot, chopped
¼ teaspoon grated fresh ginger
2 teaspoons chopped fresh coriander
1 teaspoon cornflour
1 tablespoon water, extra

Blend or process pork until finely minced. Combine pork, chopped chestnuts, shallots, garlic, celery, carrot, sauce and cornflour in a large bowl; mix well.

Add cabbage and chives to a large saucepan of boiling water, boil 2 minutes, uncovered, or until cabbage is just tender; drain, cool.

Remove and discard hard centre from cabbage leaves, cut leaves in half. Divide pork mixture evenly between leaves, fold sides in, roll up, tie with chives. Place rolls in steamer, seam side down, cover, steam for about 10 minutes (or microwave, covered, on HIGH for about 5 minutes) or until pork is tender.

Coriander Sauce: Combine water, stock cube, shallot, ginger and coriander in a small saucepan, bring to the boil, reduce heat, simmer, uncovered, for 2 minutes. Stir in blended cornflour and extra water, stir constantly over heat until sauce boils and thickens.

Serves 4.

Approximately 670 kilojoules (160 calories) per serve.

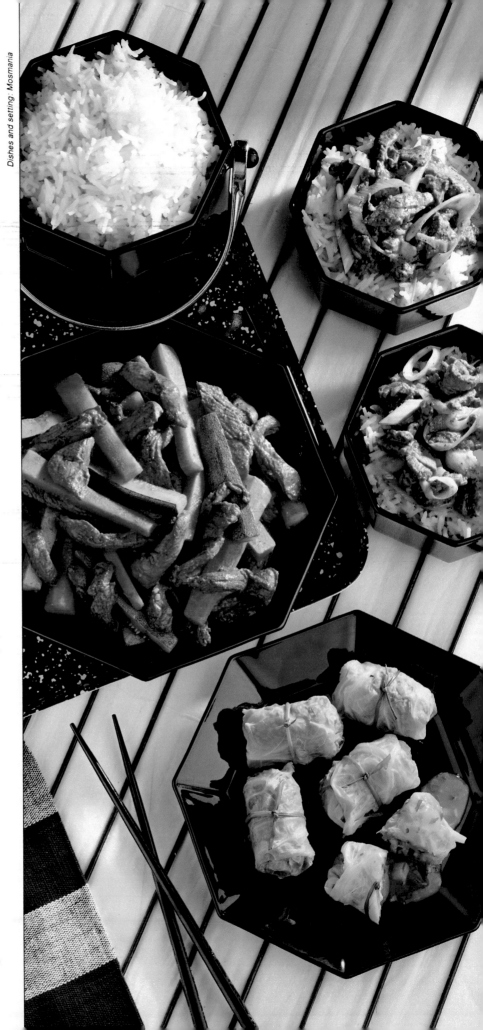

LEFT: Pork Steaks with Green Peppercorn Sauce. RIGHT: Clockwise from left: Stir-Fried Pork and Vegetables; Pork in Black Bean Sauce; Cabbage Pork Rolls

Dishes and setting: Mosmania

SIDE DISHES

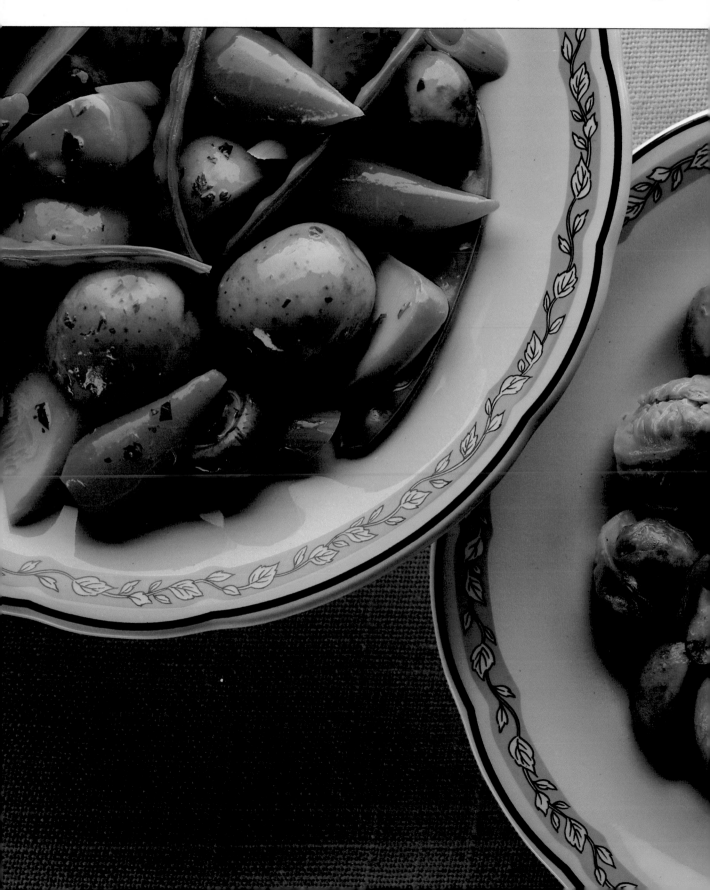

You can add plenty of flavour, interest and variety to main courses by choosing a side dish, hot or cold, that fits in with your kilojoule allowance. And these are all so wonderfully good for health and energy! Most of the recipes are also ideal for non-meat eaters.

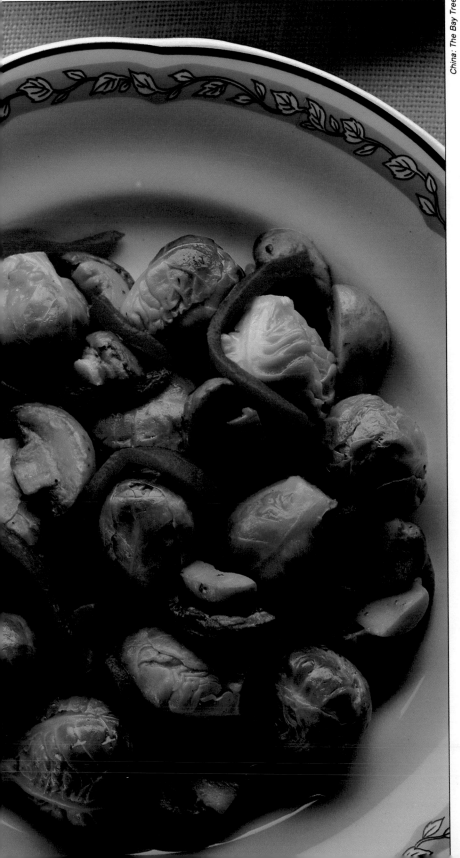

China: The Bay Tree

HOT BABY VEGETABLES WITH LEMON DRESSING

This recipe is not suitable to freeze.

20 baby carrots (180g)
6 baby new potatoes (180g)
6 baby squash (180g), sliced
180g baby mushrooms
180g snow peas
10 green shallots, sliced
30g butter, melted
1 clove garlic, crushed
1 tablespoon lemon juice
1 tablespoon chopped fresh parsley
1 tablespoon chopped fresh mint

Boil, steam or microwave all vegetables until just tender. Toss vegetables together in serving bowl; top with combined hot butter, garlic, lemon juice, parsley and mint.

Serves 4.

Approximately 575 kilojoules (137 calories) per serve.

BRUSSELS SPROUTS WITH MUSHROOMS AND PIMIENTO

Recipe unsuitable to freeze.

500g Brussels sprouts
30g butter
1 clove garlic, crushed
250g baby mushrooms, halved
1 tablespoon lemon juice
1 drained canned pimiento (60g), sliced

Boil, steam or microwave sprouts until just tender. Heat butter in frying pan, add garlic and mushrooms, cook, stirring, until mushrooms are tender. Add lemon juice, then sprouts, place in serving dish, add pimiento.

Serves 4.

Approximately 420 kilojoules (100 calories) per serve.

Top: Hot Baby Vegetables with Lemon Dressing; bottom: Brussels Sprouts with Mushrooms and Pimiento

MINTED CABBAGE SALAD

Recipe unsuitable to freeze.

3 cups shredded cabbage (250g)
1 medium red pepper (150g),
   chopped
3 green shallots, chopped
1 medium carrot (120g), chopped
DRESSING
1 teaspoon sugar
½ teaspoon grated fresh ginger
¼ cup lemon juice
1 clove garlic, crushed
1 tablespoon chopped fresh mint

Combine all ingredients in large bowl, add dressing just before serving.

Dressing: Combine all ingredients in screw-top jar, shake well.

   Serves 4.

Approximately 165 kilojoules (39 calories) per serve.

MIXED VEGETABLE STIR-FRY

This recipe is not suitable to freeze or microwave.

⅓ cup water
1 teaspoon sesame oil
1 small red pepper (100g), chopped
1 clove garlic, crushed
250g baby mushrooms, sliced
1 cup shredded cabbage (80g)
1½ cups bean sprouts (90g)
4 green shallots, chopped
2 teaspoons light soya sauce

Combine water, sesame oil, pepper and garlic in a frying pan or wok, bring to the boil, cook 1 minute. Add mushrooms, cabbage and sprouts, stir constantly over heat until vegetables are just tender. Add shallots and soya sauce, stir until heated through.
   Serves 4.

Approximately 160 kilojoules (38 calories) per serve.

Minted Cabbage Salad

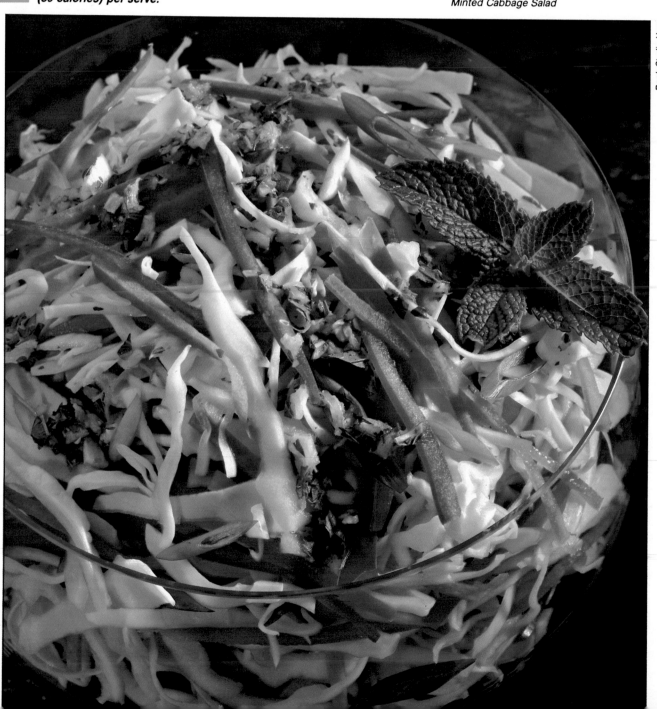

SESAME GREEN BEAN STIR-FRY

This recipe is not suitable to freeze or microwave.

185g green beans
½ x 425g can baby corn, drained
2 teaspoons oil
1 teaspoon sesame oil
2 large sticks celery (200g), sliced
1 large red pepper (225g), sliced
1 clove garlic, crushed
2 teaspoons sesame seeds
1 tablespoon light soya sauce
2 teaspoons lemon juice

Top and tail beans, cut corn into quarters lengthways. Heat oils in frying pan or wok, add vegetables, garlic and sesame seeds, stir constantly over heat for about 2 minutes or until vegetables are just tender. Add soya sauce and lemon juice, stir over heat further minute.

Serves 4.

Approximately 550 kilojoules (131 calories) per serve.

HOT MINTED TOMATO AND CUCUMBER SALAD

This recipe is not suitable to freeze or microwave.

1 medium cucumber (280g), thinly sliced
3 medium tomatoes (300g), thinly sliced
2 teaspoons oil
1 tablespoon lemon juice
1 clove garlic, crushed
1 tablespoon chopped fresh parsley
1 tablespoon grated parmesan cheese
1 tablespoon chopped fresh mint

Alternate cucumber and tomato in flameproof dish. Combine oil, lemon juice, garlic and parsley in screw-top jar, shake well, pour over tomato and cucumber. Sprinkle with cheese, grill until cheese is melted. Sprinkle with mint before serving.

Serves 4.

Approximately 220 kilojoules (53 calories) per serve.

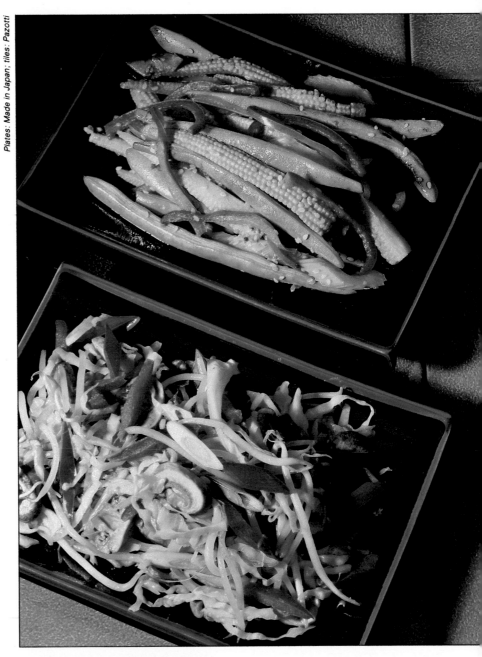

Plates: Made in Japan; tiles: Pazotti

ABOVE: Top: Sesame Green Bean Stir-Fry; bottom: Mixed Vegetable Stir-Fry.
BELOW: Hot Minted Tomato and Cucumber Salad

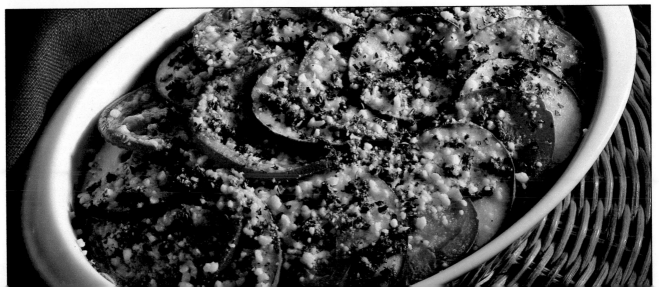

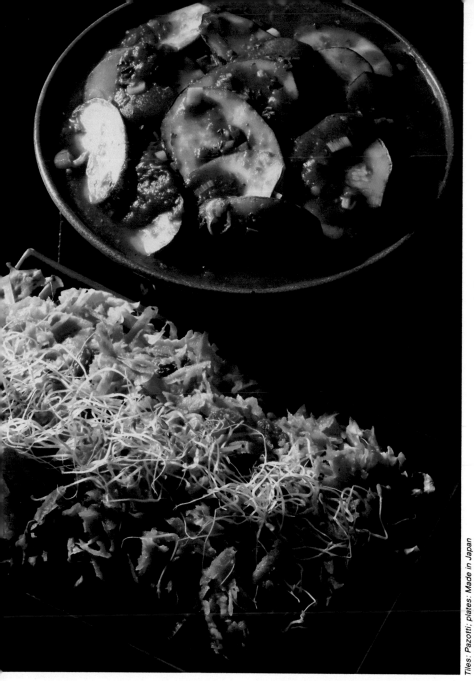

CONTINENTAL SALAD

A tasty cheese can be substituted for Jarlsberg, if preferred. Recipe unsuitable to freeze.

8 mignonette lettuce leaves
80g Jarlsberg cheese, chopped
4 slices Polish salami (40g)
3 medium gherkins (90g), sliced
3 green shallots, sliced
1 small red pepper (100g), chopped
2 tablespoons No Oil French
**   dressing**

Line bowl with lettuce, add cheese, salami, gherkins, shallots and pepper; top with dressing just before serving.
    Serves 4.

Approximately 435 kilojoules (105 calories) per serve.

ZESTY BEETROOT SALAD WITH YOGHURT DRESSING

Recipe is unsuitable to freeze.

3 large beetroot (500g)
1 large carrot (200g), coarsely grated
6 spring onions (200g), thinly sliced
1 medium stick celery (80g), thinly
**   sliced**
1 tablespoon chopped fresh parsley
½ cup alfalfa sprouts (20g)
YOGHURT DRESSING
200g carton low-fat plain yoghurt
2 teaspoons sugar
1 teaspoon lemon juice

Boil, steam or microwave beetroot until tender; drain. Cool beetroot, remove skin, chop beetroot into cubes. Combine beetroot, carrot, onions, celery and parsley in bowl. Pour dressing over salad just before serving, sprinkle with alfalfa sprouts.
    Yoghurt Dressing: Combine yoghurt, sugar and lemon juice.
    Serves 4.

Approximately 455 kilojoules (109 calories) per serve.

Tiles: Pazotti; plates: Made in Japan

ZUCCHINI TOMATO CASSEROLE

Recipe unsuitable to freeze.

15g butter
6 green shallots, chopped
1 clove garlic, crushed
5 small zucchini (500g), thickly sliced
425g can tomatoes
2 tablespoons tomato paste
2 tablespoons chopped fresh parsley
1 bay leaf

Melt butter in a saucepan, add shallots and garlic, stir constantly over heat about 3 minutes (or microwave on HIGH for about 1 minute). Stir in zucchini, undrained, crushed tomatoes, tomato paste, parsley and bay leaf. Bring to the boil, reduce heat, simmer, uncovered, 5 minutes (or microwave on HIGH for about 2 minutes). Remove bay leaf before serving.
    Serves 4.

Approximately 295 kilojoules (71 calories) per serve.

HONEYED GINGER CARROTS

Recipe unsuitable to freeze.

3 medium carrots (360g), coarsely
**   grated**
¼ cup sultanas (40g)
2 teaspoons oil
1 tablespoon lemon juice
1 tablespoon water
2 teaspoons grated fresh ginger
2 teaspoons honey
4 lettuce leaves
½ cup alfalfa sprouts (20g)

Combine carrots with sultanas in bowl. Combine oil, lemon juice, water, ginger and honey in a screw-top jar, shake well. Pour dressing over carrots and sultanas just before serving. Serve with lettuce topped with sprouts.
    Serves 4.

Approximately 345 kilojoules (82 calories) per serve.

ABOVE: Top: Zucchini Tomato Casserole; bottom: Honeyed Ginger Carrots. RIGHT: Top: Continental Salad; bottom: Zesty Beetroot Salad with Yoghurt Dressing

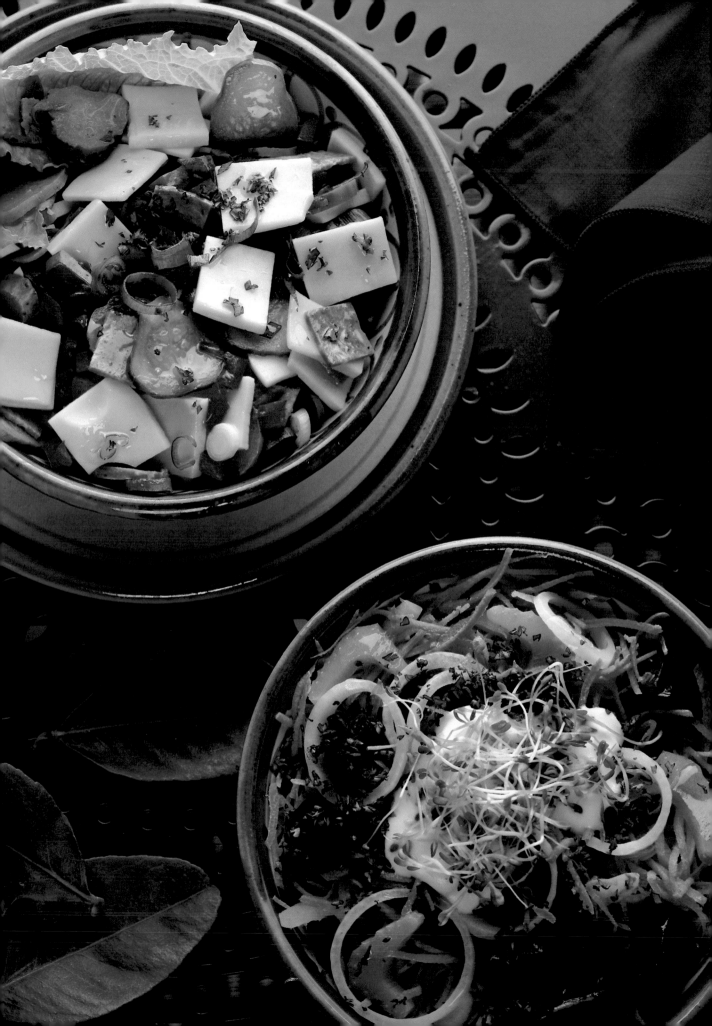

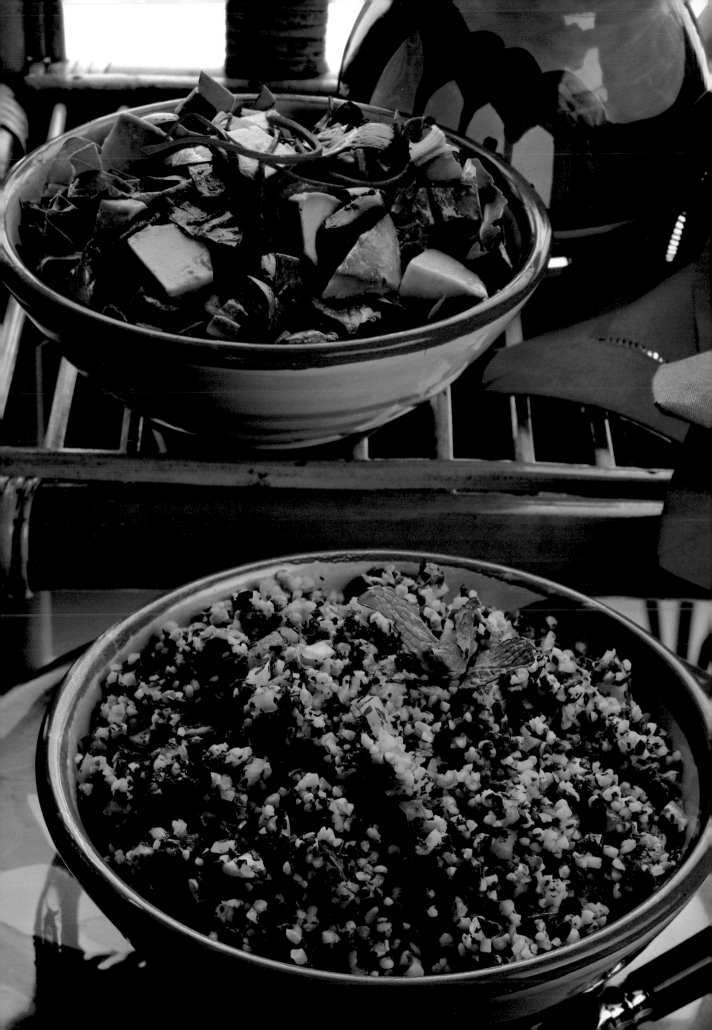

CRUNCHY SPINACH AND AVOCADO SALAD

English spinach has soft, velvety leaves, but, if this is not available, young silver beet leaves can be substituted (see Glossary, page 124). This recipe is not suitable to freeze.

40 English spinach leaves
1 avocado (200g), sliced
12 pitted black olives (50g), quartered
2 teaspoons olive oil
1 tablespoon lemon juice
1 clove garlic, crushed

Remove white stalks from spinach leaves, slice leaves into bite-size pieces. Combine spinach, avocado and olives in bowl, add combined oil, lemon juice and garlic.

Serves 4.

Approximately 930 kilojoules (222 calories) per serve.

TABBOULEH

Continental parsley is the flat-leafed variety but, if this is not available, ordinary parsley can be substituted. This recipe will keep, covered and refrigerated, for 3 days. This recipe is not suitable to freeze.

½ cup burghul (cracked wheat) (90g)
2 small tomatoes (120g), peeled, chopped
3 green shallots, chopped
1 small onion (80g), finely chopped
1 cup chopped fresh Continental parsley
½ cup chopped fresh mint
2 teaspoons oil
¼ cup lemon juice
pinch chilli powder

Cover burghul with boiling water, stand 15 minutes, drain well; rinse well under cold water, drain, blot excess moisture between pieces of absorbent paper.

Combine burghul, tomatoes, shallots, onion, parsley, mint, oil, lemon juice and chilli powder in bowl.

Serves 4.

Approximately 500 kilojoules (120 calories) per serve.

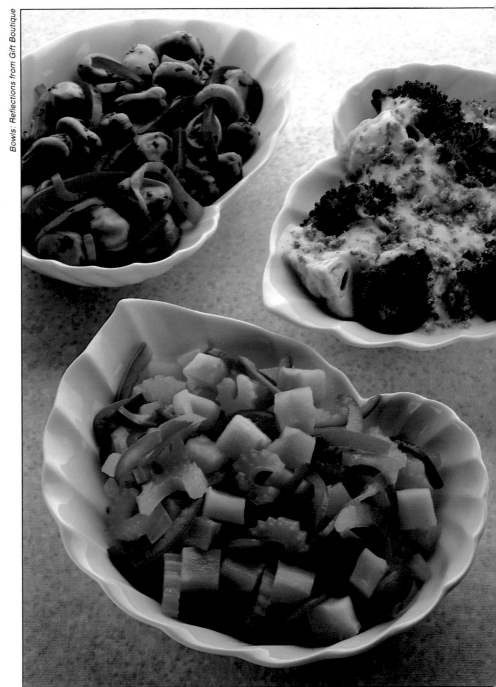

Bowls: Reflections from Gift Boutique

LEFT: Top: Crunchy Spinach and Avocado Salad; bottom: Tabbouleh. ABOVE: Clockwise from top: Broad Beans with Basil; Broccoli and Cauliflower with Cheese Sauce; Crunchy Parsnip Salad

BROAD BEANS WITH BASIL

This recipe is not suitable to freeze or microwave.

1kg fresh broad beans, shelled
15g butter
1 clove garlic, crushed
1 medium onion (120g), sliced
1 small red pepper (100g), sliced
2 tablespoons chopped fresh basil

Boil, steam or microwave beans until tender; drain. Melt butter in saucepan, add garlic and onion, stir over heat until onion is soft, add beans and pepper, stir constantly over heat for about 1 minute. Stir in basil.

Serves 4.

Approximately 335 kilojoules (80 calories) per serve.

CRUNCHY PARSNIP SALAD

Recipe unsuitable to freeze.

3 large parsnips (700g), chopped
1 medium onion (120g), chopped
2 medium sticks celery (160g), chopped
1 small red pepper (100g), finely chopped
2 teaspoons sugar
1 tablespoon lemon juice
¼ cup water

Boil, steam or microwave parsnips until tender, drain. Cook onion, celery and pepper in saucepan with sugar, lemon juice and water until onion is soft, pour over parsnips, serve hot or cold.

Serves 4.

Approximately 470 kilojoules (112 calories) per serve.

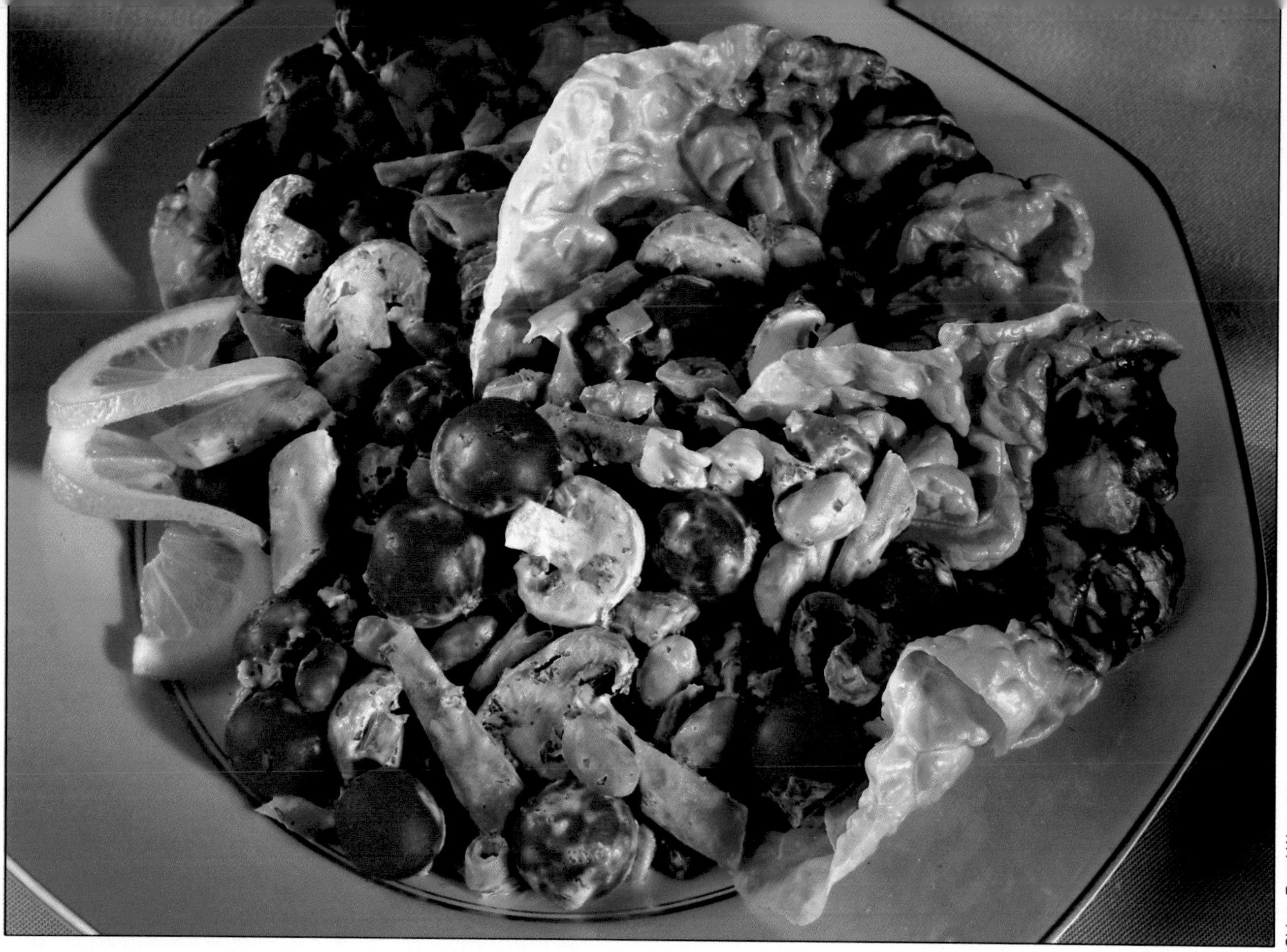

China: Royal Worcester

BROCCOLI AND CAULIFLOWER WITH CHEESE SAUCE

Recipe unsuitable to freeze.

250g broccoli
250g cauliflower
15g butter
3 teaspoons plain flour
1 cup skim milk
¼ cup grated tasty cheese (30g)
2 green shallots, chopped
1 tablespoon chopped fresh parsley
¼ cup stale wholemeal breadcrumbs
pinch paprika

Cut broccoli and cauliflower into flowerets, boil, steam or microwave until tender; drain, place in a shallow ovenproof dish.

Melt butter in a saucepan, stir in flour, cook 1 minute (or microwave on HIGH about 1 minute). Stir in milk, stir constantly over heat until mixture boils and thickens (or microwave on HIGH about 3 minutes). Remove from heat, add cheese, shallots and parsley, stir until cheese is melted.

Pour sauce over vegetables, top with combined breadcrumbs and paprika. Bake in moderate oven 20 minutes or until heated through (or microwave on HIGH about 5 minutes).

Serves 4.

Approximately 520 kilojoules (124 calories) per serve.

MUSHROOM AND GREEN BEAN SALAD WITH SOUR CREAM

Add dressing just before serving. This recipe is not suitable to freeze.

200g green beans
250g baby mushrooms, halved
½ x 300g can three-bean mix, rinsed, drained
4 green shallots, thinly sliced
250g punnet cherry tomatoes

DRESSING

2 tablespoons No Oil French dressing
1 tablespoon sour light cream
1 tablespoon chopped fresh parsley
1 teaspoon grated lemon rind

Top and tail beans, cut into 2cm lengths. Boil, steam or microwave beans until just tender, drain, rinse under cold water, drain. Combine beans with remaining ingredients, add dressing, toss well.

Dressing: Combine all ingredients in small bowl, mix well.

Serves 4.

Approximately 315 kilojoules (75 calories) per serve.

ABOVE: Mushroom and Green Bean Salad with Sour Cream. RIGHT: Top: Marinated Green Beans; bottom: Minted Orange Potatoes

MARINATED GREEN BEANS

Recipe unsuitable to freeze.

500g green beans
⅓ cup No Oil French dressing
2 cloves garlic, crushed
1 drained canned pimiento (60g), chopped
2 medium gherkins (60g), chopped

Top and tail beans. Boil, steam or microwave beans until just tender; drain, rinse under cold water. Combine dressing, garlic, pimiento and gherkins in a screw-top jar, shake well; pour over beans, marinate 1 hour in refrigerator before serving.

Serves 4.

Approximately 90 kilojoules (22 calories) per serve.

MINTED ORANGE POTATOES

Recipe is unsuitable to freeze.

750g baby new potatoes
15g butter
2 teaspoons grated orange rind
¼ cup orange juice
¼ cup grated parmesan cheese (20g)
2 tablespoons chopped fresh mint

Boil, steam or microwave potatoes until tender, drain. Heat butter in frying pan, add potatoes, toss gently over heat until potatoes are browned all over. Stir in orange rind, juice, cheese and mint.

Serves 4.

Approximately 865 kilojoules (206 calories) per serve.

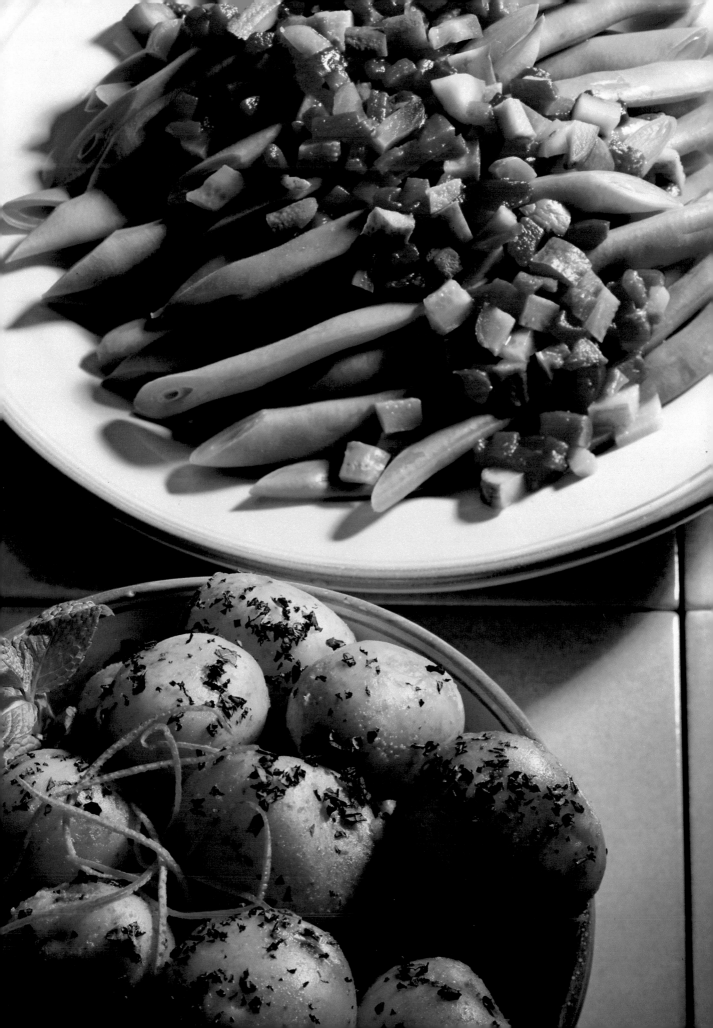

RADICCHIO AND FENNEL SALAD

Witlof is also known as Belgian endive and chicory. Its small leaves have a slightly bitter taste. Recipe unsuitable to freeze or microwave.

1 radicchio lettuce
1 witlof (chicory)
1 medium fennel bulb (300g), thinly
**   sliced**
40 English spinach leaves, sliced
8 radishes (160g), chopped
1 small fresh red chilli, finely
**   chopped**
2 green shallots, chopped
½ cup No Oil Italian dressing

Break lettuce and witlof into separate leaves, combine with fennel, spinach and radishes in bowl. Add the combined chilli, shallots and dressing just before serving.

Serves 4.

Approximately 200 kilojoules (48 calories) per serve.

MUSHROOM AND HERB SALAD

Unsuitable to freeze or microwave.

375g baby mushrooms
2 tablespoons chopped fresh parsley
2 teaspoons chopped fresh chives
1 tablespoon oil
2 cloves garlic, crushed
¼ cup lemon juice
¼ teaspoon ground coriander
¼ teaspoon cayenne pepper

Combine mushrooms, parsley and chives in a bowl. Heat oil in a small frying pan, add garlic, cook until lightly browned, stir in lemon juice, coriander and cayenne pepper, pour over mushroom mixture, refrigerate several hours before serving.

Serves 4.

Approximately 255 kilojoules (60 calories) per serve.

POTATO AND BRUSSELS SPROUTS SALAD

Recipe unsuitable to freeze.

500g baby new potatoes
200g baby Brussels sprouts
1 medium red pepper (150g), sliced
FRESH OREGANO DRESSING
2 tablespoons low oil coleslaw
**   dressing**
1 tablespoon chopped fresh chives
1 tablespoon chopped fresh oregano

Boil, steam or microwave unpeeled potatoes until tender; drain. Place in bowl of iced water. Boil, steam or microwave sprouts until just tender; drain, place into a bowl of iced water; drain well.

Combine potatoes, sprouts and pepper in bowl, add dressing just before serving.

Fresh Oregano Dressing: Combine all ingredients; mix well.

Serves 4.

Approximately 520 kilojoules (124 calories) per serve.

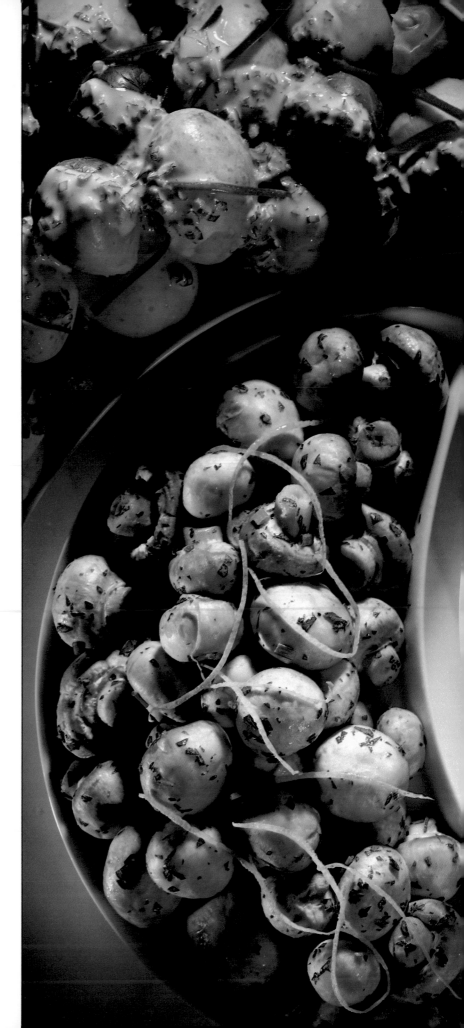

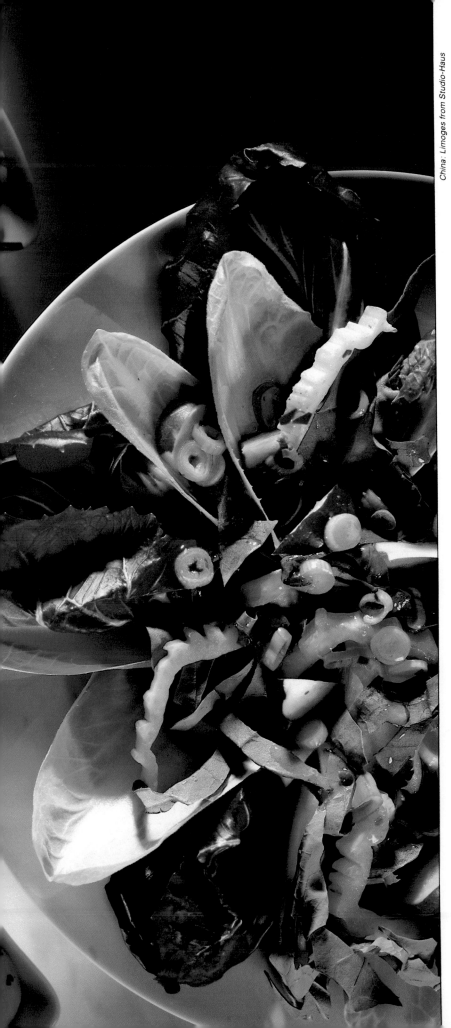

CRISPY CHINESE CABBAGE STIR-FRY

Dried mushrooms are available from Asian stores. Recipe unsuitable to freeze or microwave.

6 dried mushrooms
125g snow peas
2 teaspoons oil
1 medium onion (120g), chopped
1 medium carrot (120g), sliced
1 medium red pepper (150g), chopped
230g can sliced water chestnuts, drained
2 small chicken stock cubes, crumbled
¾ cup water
1 tablespoon light soya sauce
4 medium sticks celery (320g), sliced
4 green shallots, chopped
4 cups bean sprouts (250g)
1 small Chinese cabbage, sliced

Cover mushrooms with boiling water, stand 20 minutes, drain, remove and discard stems, slice mushrooms thinly. Top and tail snow peas.

Heat oil in a wok or large frying pan. Add onion, stir-fry 1 minute. Add carrot, pepper and water chestnuts, stir-fry 1 minute. Add combined stock cubes, water and soya sauce, bring to the boil, add celery, snow peas, shallots, sprouts, cabbage and mushrooms, stir-fry 1 minute.

Serves 4.

Approximately 600 kilojoules (143 calories) per serve.

CAULIFLOWER AND FRESH HERB SALAD

Make this salad as close to serving time as possible. This recipe is not suitable to freeze.

500g cauliflower
1 tablespoon chopped fresh basil
1 tablespoon chopped fresh mint
1 tablespoon chopped fresh parsley
2 tablespoons orange juice
2 tablespoons lemon juice

Cut cauliflower into flowerets. Boil, steam or microwave cauliflower until just tender; drain, cool.

Combine cauliflower, basil, mint and parsley in bowl, top with juices just before serving.

Serves 4.

Approximately 100 kilojoules (24 calories) per serve.

Clockwise: Radicchio and Fennel Salad; Mushroom and Herb Salad; Potato and Brussels Sprouts Salad

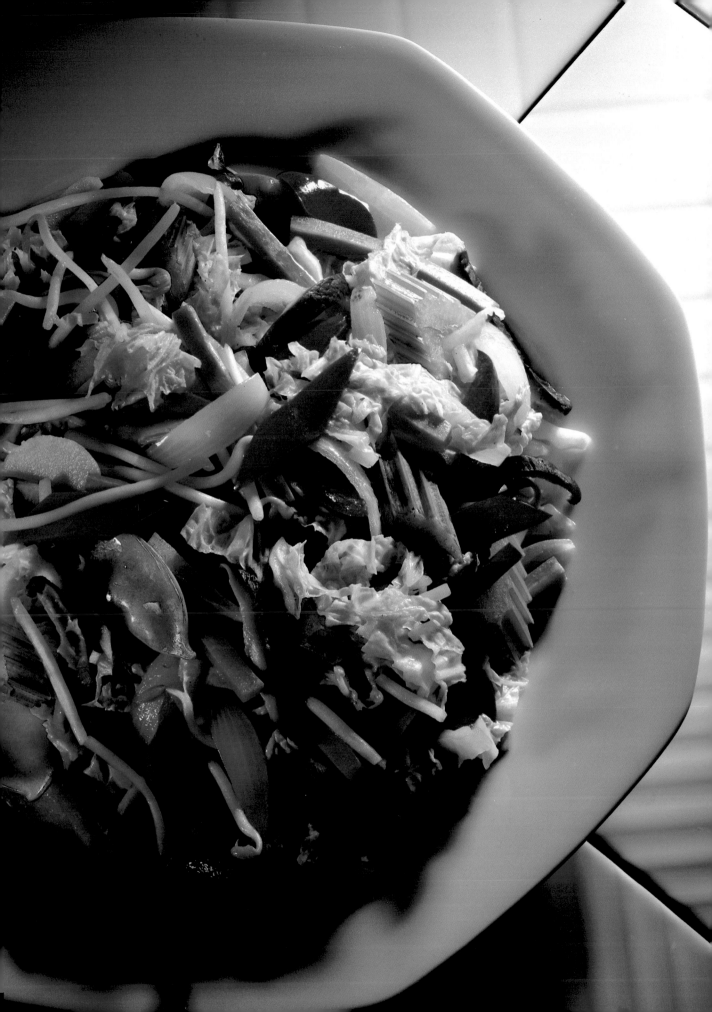

CHEESE AND GHERKIN POTATOES

We used red-skinned potatoes in this recipe. This dish is not suitable to freeze.

2 large potatoes (370g)
½ cup low-fat cottage cheese (120g)
2 medium gherkins (60g), finely chopped
1 tablespoon chopped fresh chives
pinch chilli powder

Place potatoes in ovenproof dish, bake in moderate oven for about 1 hour or until potatoes are tender (or microwave on HIGH for about 8 minutes).

Cut potatoes in half, scoop out centres, put shells aside. Place potato in bowl, mash well, stir in cottage cheese, gherkins and chives. Spoon mixture back into potato shells, sprinkle each with a little chilli powder. Bake in moderate oven further 10 minutes (or microwave on HIGH for about 3 minutes) or until heated through.

Serves 4.

Approximately 455 kilojoules (109 calories) per serve.

TOMATOES WITH RICE AND ZUCCHINI

You will need to cook 2 tablespoons of rice for this recipe. The dish is not suitable to freeze or microwave.

4 large tomatoes (700g)
1 tablespoon tomato paste
1 clove garlic, crushed
½ teaspoon dried basil leaves
1 small zucchini (100g), grated
½ cup cooked rice
½ cup grated tasty cheese (60g)

Cut tops from tomatoes, scoop out flesh, put shells aside. Chop flesh roughly, combine in saucepan with tomato paste, garlic and basil. Bring to the boil, boil rapidly, uncovered, until almost all the liquid has evaporated. Stir in zucchini, rice and half the cheese. Fill tomatoes with mixture, top with remaining cheese, bake in moderate oven 10 minutes or until cheese is melted.

Serves 4.

Approximately 565 kilojoules (135 calories) per serve.

BELOW: Left: Tomatoes with Rice and Zucchini; right: Cheese and Gherkin Potatoes. RIGHT: Cauliflower and Fresh Herb Salad. LEFT: Crispy Chinese Cabbage Stir-Fry

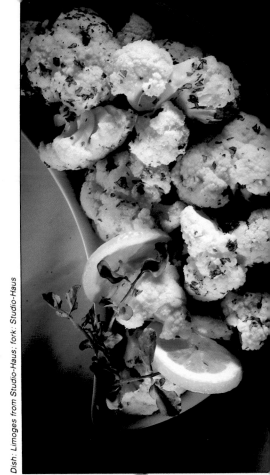

Dish: Limoges from Studio-Haus; fork: Studio-Haus

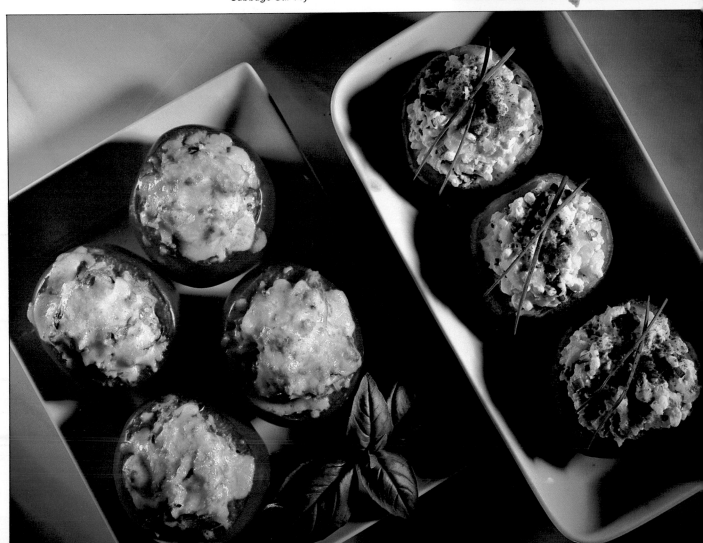

DESSERTS

Spoil yourself with one of our delicious hot desserts or a cool, fruity, luscious treat. These, with our special ice-cream and ices, are among the tempting sweets you'll never believe could be so low in kilojoules per serve. We have used mostly liquid and powdered sweeteners, see the Glossary on page 124 for further information.

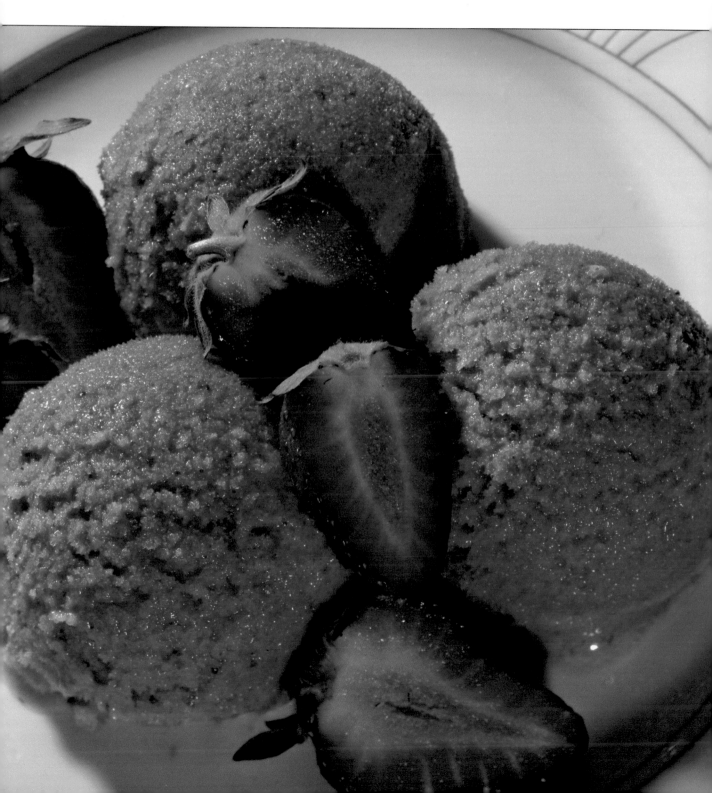

BRANDIED STRAWBERRY AND YOGHURT SORBET

Sorbet can be made up to 3 days ahead; keep, covered, in freezer.

½ cup sugar (125g)
½ cup water
1 tablespoon brandy
250g punnet strawberries
200g carton low-fat plain yoghurt
1 egg white

Combine sugar, water and brandy in saucepan, stir constantly over heat, without boiling, until sugar is dissolved. Bring to the boil, reduce heat, simmer, uncovered, without stirring for 5 minutes or until mixture is thick. Cool sugar syrup to room temperature; refrigerate until cold.

Blend or process strawberries and yoghurt until smooth, add sugar syrup, process until combined. Pour mixture into lamington pan, cover with foil, freeze several hours or until set.

Break up mixture using a fork, fold in firmly beaten egg white. Return mixture to pan, cover, freeze several hours or until set.

Serves 4.

■ *Approximately 720 kilojoules (172 calories) per serve.*

YOGHURT PASSIONFRUIT ICE-CREAM

Ice-cream can be made up to 3 days ahead; keep covered tightly with foil in freezer. Recipe makes about 10 half cup serves.

¼ cup honey
2 x 200g cartons low-fat plain yoghurt
2 teaspoons gelatine
1 tablespoon water
2 egg whites
2 medium passionfruit

Combine honey and yoghurt in bowl, stir until smooth. Sprinkle gelatine over water, dissolve over hot water (or microwave on HIGH about 20 seconds), cool, do not allow to set; stir into yoghurt mixture. Spread into lamington pan, cover with foil, freeze for about 2 hours or until the mixture has set.

Transfer yoghurt mixture to small bowl of electric mixer, beat until mixture thickens and doubles in bulk, transfer to large bowl. Beat egg whites until firm peaks form, gently fold egg whites and passionfruit into the yoghurt mixture. Pour back into lamington pan, cover, freeze for about 3 hours or until set.

Makes about 1¼ litres (5 cups).

■ *Approximately 215 kilojoules (50 calories) per serve.*

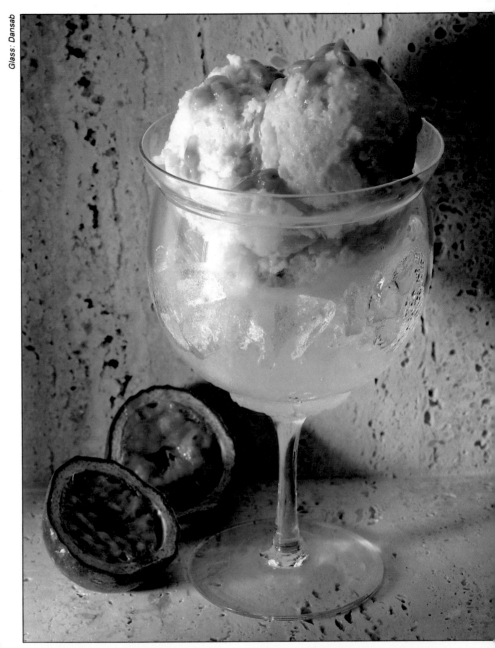

LEFT: Brandied Strawberry and Yoghurt Sorbet. ABOVE: Yoghurt Passionfruit Ice-Cream

Glass: Dansab

STRAWBERRY HAZELNUT CAKE

This cake is deliciously special and will serve 10 slimmers. This recipe is not suitable to freeze or microwave.

4 eggs
¼ cup castor sugar (60g)
⅓ cup self-raising flour (50g)
⅓ cup ground hazelnuts (40g)
STRAWBERRY FILLING
1 cup ricotta cheese (200g)
1 tablespoon low kilojoule strawberry jam
250g punnet strawberries
RICOTTA CREAM
⅔ cup ricotta cheese (125g)
⅓ cup cream
1 teaspoon vanilla essence

Grease a deep 20cm round cake pan; line base with baking or greaseproof paper, lightly grease paper.

Beat eggs and sugar in small bowl with electric mixer until thick and creamy. Fold in sifted flour and hazelnuts; pour mixture into prepared pan. Bake in moderate oven for about 30 minutes, turn onto wire rack to cool.

When cake is cold, cut in half horizontally. Place half the cake on serving plate, spread with filling, top with remaining cake. Spread ricotta cream over cake, decorate with reserved strawberries and ground hazelnuts. Refrigerate several hours.

Strawberry Filling: Blend or process cheese, jam and half the strawberries until smooth; reserve remaining strawberries for decoration.

Ricotta Cream: Blend or process all ingredients until smooth.

■ *Approximately 720 kilojoules (172 calories) per serve.*

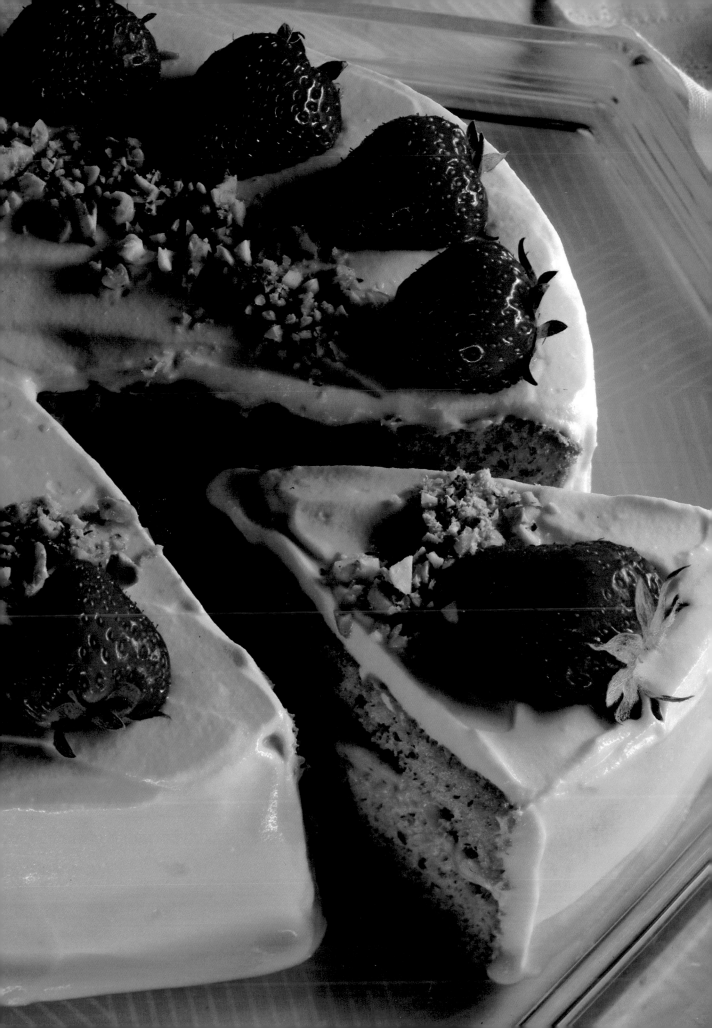

FRUITY COCONUT YOGHURT RICE CREAM

Recipe can be made up to 2 days ahead; keep, covered, in refrigerator. This recipe is not suitable to freeze or microwave.

⅓ cup rice (75g)
180ml can coconut milk
½ cup low-fat plain yoghurt
1 tablespoon castor sugar
1 medium banana (150g), thinly sliced
2 medium passionfruit

Add rice gradually to saucepan of boiling water, boil rapidly, uncovered, for 10 minutes or until just tender, drain. Rinse rice under cold water, drain well.

Combine rice, coconut milk, yoghurt, sugar, banana and passionfruit pulp in bowl, place into 4 serving dishes; refrigerate several hours before serving.

Serves 4.

Approximately 1050 kilojoules (250 calories) per serve.

APRICOT ORANGE CREMES

Recipe unsuitable to freeze.

⅓ cup flaked almonds (30g)
425g can unsweetened apricot halves
¾ cup ricotta cheese (150g)
2 teaspoons sugar
1 teaspoon grated orange rind
1 tablespoon orange juice
ORANGE SAUCE
1 teaspoon cornflour
2 tablespoons orange juice
1 teaspoon sugar

Toast almonds on an oven tray in moderate oven for 5 minutes.

Drain apricots well, reserve half cup juice. Beat cheese, sugar, rind and juice together in bowl until well combined. Fill apricot halves with creamy cheese mixture, serve topped with sauce and almonds.

Orange Sauce: Combine blended cornflour and orange juice in saucepan, stir in sugar and reserved apricot juice, stir constantly over heat until sauce boils and thickens (or microwave on HIGH for about 1 minute).

Serves 4.

Approximately 645 kilojoules (154 calories) per serve.

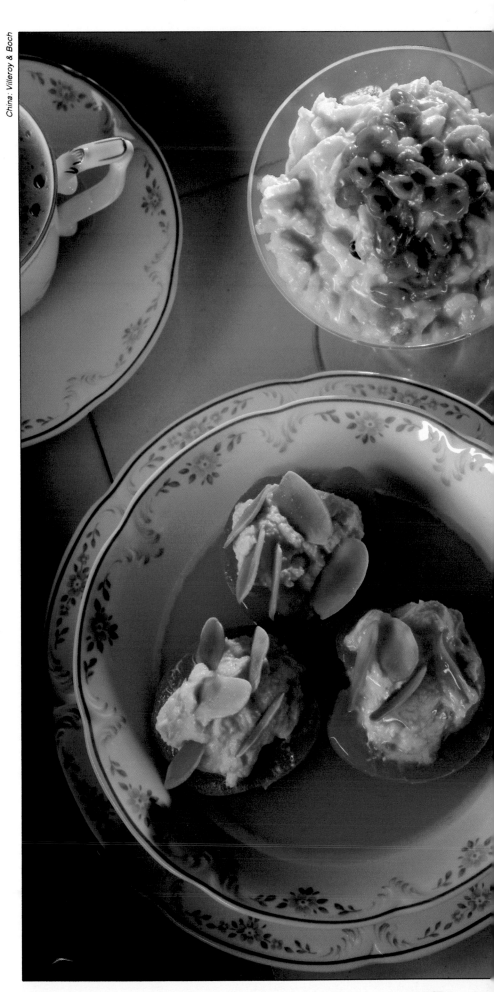

China: Villeroy & Boch

LEFT: Strawberry Hazelnut Cake. RIGHT: Top: Fruity Coconut Yoghurt Rice Cream; bottom: Apricot Orange Cremes

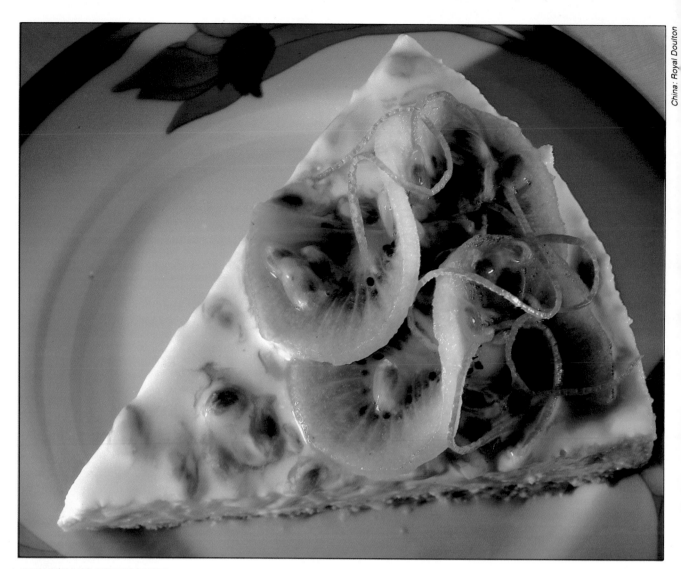

CREAMY PASSIONFRUIT CHEESECAKE

Cheesecake can be made up to 2 days ahead; keep, covered, in refrigerator. Spread topping on cheesecake just before serving. Cheesecake will cut into about 10 slices. This recipe is not suitable to freeze.

1 cup sweet biscuit crumbs (125g)
30g butter, melted
2 teaspoons water
FILLING
9g sachet low kilojoule passionfruit jelly
1 cup boiling water
250g carton low-fat cottage cheese
½ cup low-fat plain yoghurt
TOPPING
¼ cup cream
¼ cup low-fat plain yoghurt
1 teaspoon sugar
2 medium passionfruit

Combine crumbs, butter and water in bowl, mix well. Press over base of 20cm springform pan, refrigerate 30 minutes. Pour filling over base, refrigerate until set. Spread with topping. Refrigerate 30 minutes before serving.
Filling: Combine jelly and water in bowl, stir until jelly is dissolved; cool to room temperature, do not allow to set. Blend or process cottage cheese and yoghurt until smooth, add jelly, process until combined.
Topping: Combine all ingredients in bowl, stir until combined.

Approximately 575 kilojoules (137 calories) per serve.

FRESH FRUIT WITH MANGO AND HONEY YOGHURT

Any fresh fruit in season can be used, but remember to adjust kilojoule count accordingly. This recipe is not suitable to freeze.

250g punnet strawberries
2 medium kiwi fruit (200g), sliced
1 cup grapes (200g)
1 medium passionfruit
1 small mango (200g)
½ cup low-fat plain yoghurt
2 teaspoons honey

Divide fruit into 4 serving dishes. Blend or process mango, yoghurt and honey until smooth, place in jug, refrigerate before serving over fruit.

Serves 4.

Approximately 510 kilojoules (122 calories) per serve.

BERRY WATERMELON SORBET

Sorbet can be made a week ahead; keep, covered, in freezer. Use fresh or frozen berries in this recipe; if mixture is not sweet enough, add artificial sweetener to taste. This recipe makes about 8 half-cup serves.

2 cups berries (250g)
4 cups watermelon chunks (1kg)
2 tablespoons castor sugar
1 tablespoon lemon juice

Blend or process berries until smooth, strain into a bowl to remove seeds. Return purée to processor with watermelon, sugar and juice, process until smooth. Pour into lamington pan, cover with foil, freeze until almost set. Return mixture to processor, process until smooth. Repeat freezing and processing once more. Cover, freeze several hours or until set.

Makes about 1 litre (4 cups).

Approximately 235 kilojoules (56 calories) per serve.

RIGHT: Top: Fresh Fruit with Mango and Honey Yoghurt; bottom: Berry Watermelon Sorbet. ABOVE: Creamy Passionfruit Cheesecake

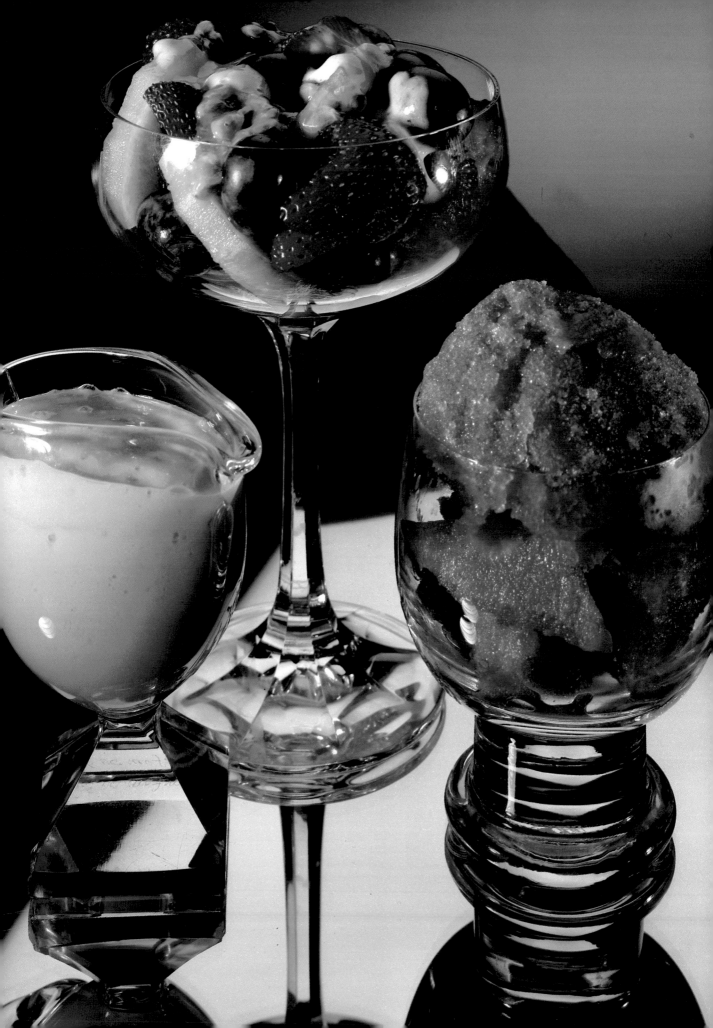

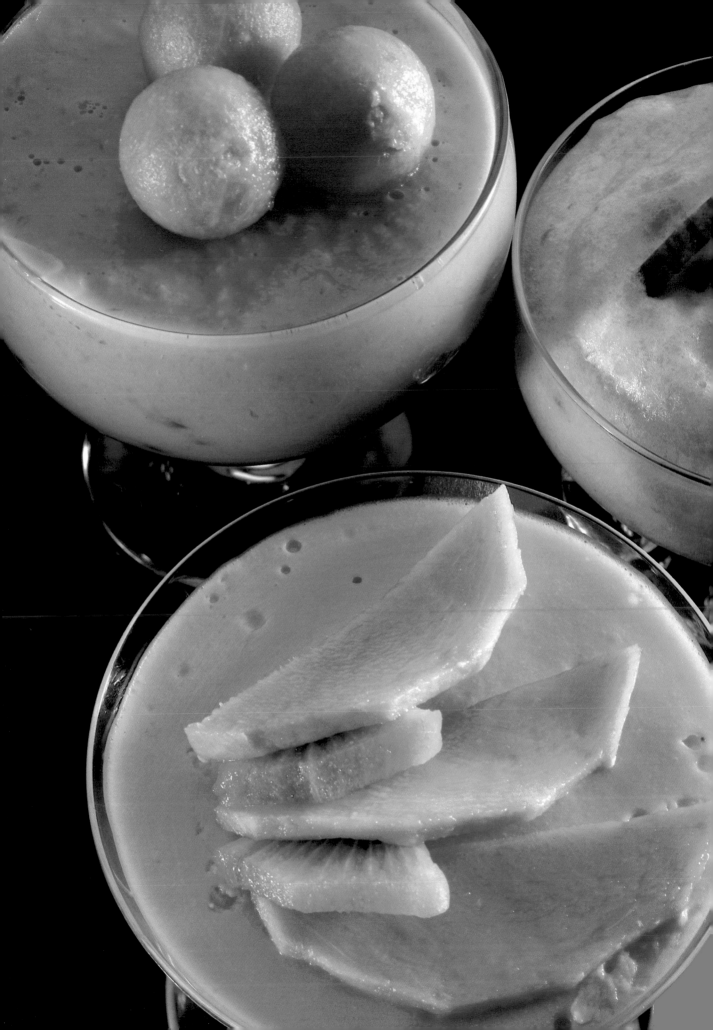

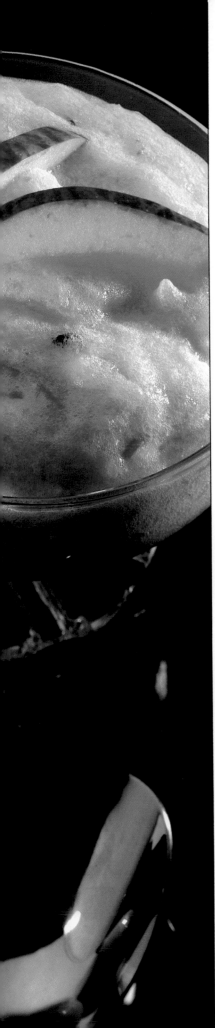

ROCKMELON PASSIONFRUIT MOUSSE

Mousse can be made up to a day ahead. You will need to buy a 1kg rockmelon. Recipe unsuitable to freeze.

5 cups chopped rockmelon (750g)
2 tablespoons honey
200g carton low-fat plain yoghurt
1 tablespoon gelatine
2 tablespoons water
2 medium passionfruit

Blend or process rockmelon, honey and yoghurt until smooth. Sprinkle gelatine over water, dissolve over hot water (or microwave on HIGH for about 20 seconds). Stir gelatine mixture and passionfruit pulp into melon mixture. Pour mixture into 4 serving dishes, refrigerate several hours or until set.
Serves 4.

 Approximately 525 kilojoules (125 calories) per serve.

CREAMY MANGO DELIGHT

Skim milk must be chilled well before whisking. Recipe unsuitable to freeze.

2 medium mangoes (480g)
2 teaspoons sugar
1 tablespoon water
2 teaspoons gelatine
2 tablespoons water, extra
¾ cup evaporated skim milk

Blend or process mangoes until smooth. Combine sugar, water and mango purée in bowl. Sprinkle gelatine over extra water, dissolve over hot water (or microwave on HIGH for about 20 seconds), add to mango mixture. Whisk milk in a bowl until frothy and fold into mango mixture. Pour into serving dishes, refrigerate until set.
Serves 4.

 Approximately 490 kilojoules (117 calories) per serve.

APPLE PASSIONFRUIT WHIP

Recipe can be prepared up to 2 days ahead; keep, covered, in refrigerator. This recipe is not suitable to freeze.

4 large apples (800g), chopped
½ cup water
2 teaspoons sugar
3 medium passionfruit
1 teaspoon grated orange rind
3 egg whites

Combine apples and water in a saucepan, bring to the boil, cover, reduce heat, simmer 5 minutes or until apples are tender. Transfer to large bowl, stir in sugar, passionfruit and orange rind, cool to room temperature.

Beat egg whites in small bowl until soft peaks form, fold into apple mixture, refrigerate 1 hour before serving.
Serves 4.

Approximately 515 kilojoules (123 calories) per serve.

FLUFFY FRUIT MOUSSE

Mousse can be made up to 2 days ahead; keep, covered, in refrigerator. This recipe is not suitable to freeze.

⅔ cup apricot nectar
⅔ cup pear juice
2 teaspoons gelatine
2 tablespoons water
2 teaspoons sugar
1 egg, separated
1 medium fresh peach (150g), sliced

Pour juices into separate small bowls.

Sprinkle gelatine over water, dissolve over hot water (or microwave on HIGH for about 20 seconds), cool to room temperature.

Combine sugar, egg yolk and gelatine mixture in bowl, divide evenly into bowls of fruit juices. Refrigerate fruit mixtures until slightly thickened (about the consistency of unbeaten egg white). Beat egg white in small bowl until soft peaks form, divide between fruit mixtures, fold in lightly. Pour mixtures simultaneously into 4 dishes (half cup capacity), refrigerate until set. Decorate with peach slices.
Serves 4.

 Approximately 375 kilojoules (90 calories) per serve.

CREAMY MOCHA MOUSSE

Mousse can be made a day ahead; keep, covered, in refrigerator. This recipe is not suitable to freeze.

375ml can evaporated skim milk
2 eggs, lightly beaten
1 tablespoon cocoa
2 teaspoons dry instant coffee
¼ teaspoon liquid sweetener
2 teaspoons gelatine
¼ cup water
¼ cup cream

Combine milk, eggs, sifted cocoa, coffee and liquid sweetener in a saucepan, beat with a rotary beater or electric mixer until smooth, stir mixture constantly over heat, without boiling, until mixture is warm.

Sprinkle gelatine over water, dissolve over hot water (or microwave on HIGH for about 20 seconds), stir into chocolate mixture with cream. Pour into 4 dishes (half cup capacity), refrigerate until set.
Serves 4.

 Approximately 725 kilojoules (173 calories) per serve.

Clockwise from top: Rockmelon Passionfruit Mousse; Apple Passionfruit Whip; Creamy Mango Delight

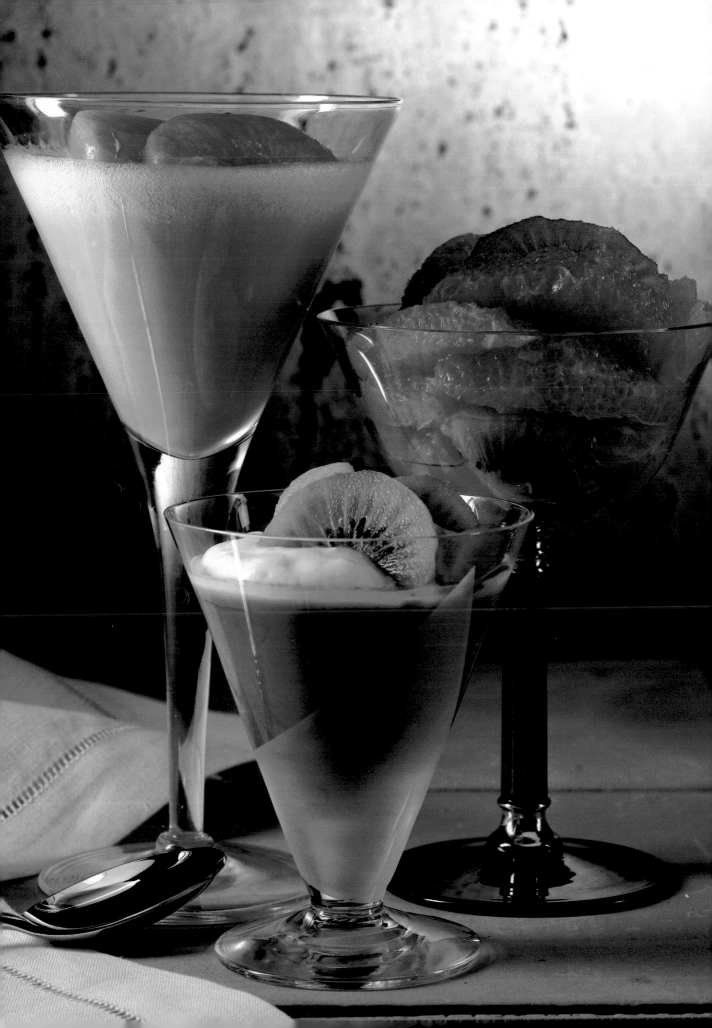

CITRUS LIQUEUR DESSERT

Grand Marnier and Cointreau are citrus-flavoured liqueurs. This recipe is not suitable to freeze.

1 medium grapefruit (390g)
3 large oranges (660g)
2 medium kiwi fruit (200g), sliced
1 teaspoon sugar
1 tablespoon Grand Marnier or Cointreau

Peel grapefruit and oranges, removing all pith and membrane, break into segments. Combine all fruit in a bowl with combined sugar and Grand Marnier, refrigerate until ready to serve.

Serves 4.

Approximately 405 kilojoules (97 calories) per serve.

ALMOND ROLL WITH LEMON CREAM

Filled roll can be prepared up to a day in advance; store, covered, in refrigerator. This cake will cut into 10 slices. Recipe is not suitable to freeze or microwave.

4 eggs
¼ teaspoon almond essence
¼ cup castor sugar (60g)
⅓ cup self-raising flour (50g)
¼ cup packaged ground almonds (30g)
LEMON CREAM
1 cup ricotta cheese (200g)
1 tablespoon sugar
2 tablespoons cream
1 teaspoon grated lemon rind
2 tablespoons lemon juice

Grease and line base of a 25cm x 30cm Swiss roll pan with baking or greaseproof paper.

Beat eggs and essence in small bowl with electric mixer until thick and creamy. Gradually add sugar, beat until sugar is dissolved. Transfer mixture to large bowl. Gently fold in sifted flour and almonds. Pour mixture into prepared pan, bake in moderate oven for about 12 minutes.

Cover cake rack with baking or greaseproof paper, spray paper with non-stick spray. Turn cake immediately onto paper, carefully remove and discard lining paper.

To roll cake, place narrow end towards you, carefully lift baking paper so the cake rolls up loosely. Stand 30 minutes, unroll, spread with lemon cream, roll up. Refrigerate 1 hour before cutting.

Lemon Cream: Beat all ingredients in bowl until smooth.

Approximately 585 kilojoules (140 calories) per serve.

LEFT: Clockwise from left: Fluffy Fruit Mousse; Citrus Liqueur Dessert; Creamy Mocha Mousse. RIGHT: Top: Almond Roll with Lemon Cream; bottom: Orange Sponge Roll

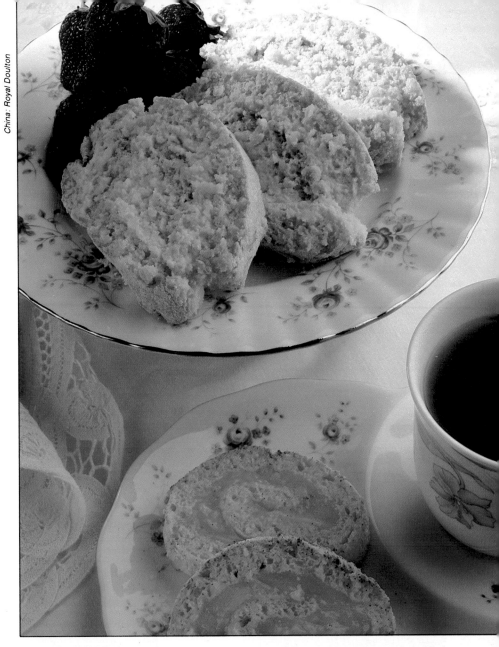

China: Royal Doulton

ORANGE SPONGE ROLL

This sponge will cut into 10 slices. It will keep, covered, in the refrigerator for up to 2 days. Recipe is not suitable to freeze or microwave.

4 egg whites
½ cup castor sugar (125g)
½ cup plain flour (75g)
1 teaspoon grated orange rind
2 teaspoons orange juice
3 tablespoons icing sugar
1 teaspoon ground cinnamon
FILLING
2 tablespoons cornflour
¼ cup castor sugar (60g)
1 teaspoon grated orange rind
⅓ cup orange juice
¾ cup water
2 egg yolks

Grease and line base of a 25cm x 30cm Swiss roll pan with baking or greaseproof paper.

Beat egg whites in small bowl with electric mixer until soft peaks form. Gradually add sugar, beat until sugar is dissolved. Transfer mixture to large bowl, fold in sifted flour, then combined rind and juice. Spread mixture into prepared pan. Bake in a slow oven for about 20 minutes or until just firm to touch. Cake will be pale in colour.

Cover a cake rack with a sheet of baking paper or greaseproof paper. Sift 2 tablespoons of the icing sugar over the paper. Turn cake onto paper, carefully remove and discard lining paper. To roll cake, place narrow end towards you, carefully lift baking paper so the cake rolls loosely. Stand for 20 minutes, unroll cake, spread filling evenly over cake, roll up. Dust with the combined remaining sifted icing sugar and cinnamon.

Filling: Combine cornflour, sugar, rind, juice and water in saucepan. Stir constantly over heat until mixture boils and thickens. Quickly stir in egg yolks, cover surface of filling with plastic wrap to prevent a skin forming, cool to room temperature; stir well before using.

Approximately 640 kilojoules (153 calories) per serve.

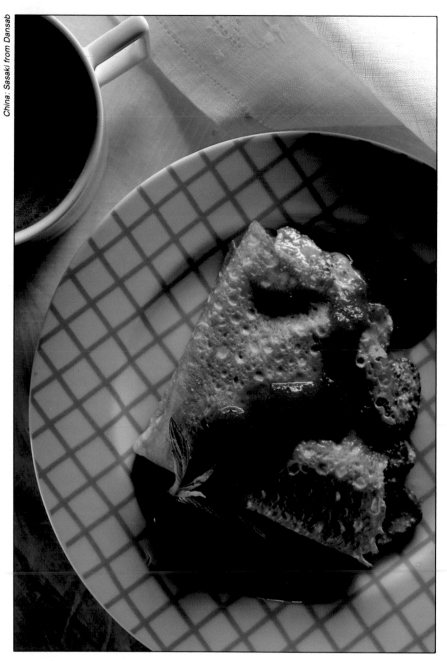

China: Sasaki from Dansab

STRAWBERRY AND ORANGE CREPES

This recipe is not suitable to freeze or microwave.

CREPE BATTER
¼ cup plain flour (40g)
1 egg, lightly beaten
½ cup skim milk
½ teaspoon oil
CREAMY STRAWBERRY FILLING
¼ cup low-fat cottage cheese (60g)
2 teaspoons sugar
½ teaspoon grated orange rind
2 teaspoons orange juice
250g punnet strawberries, sliced
STRAWBERRY ORANGE SAUCE
125g strawberries
2 teaspoons orange juice

Crepe Batter: Sift flour into bowl, make well in centre, gradually stir in combined egg, milk and oil, mix to smooth batter, allow to stand 15 minutes (or the batter can be made in a blender or processor).

Grease a heated frying pan, add quarter of the batter to pan, cook until set and lightly browned underneath. Turn crepe carefully, cook other side. Repeat with remaining batter. Divide filling between crepes, fold crepes in quarters, serve with sauce.
Creamy Strawberry Filling: Combine sieved cottage cheese, sugar, rind and juice in bowl, mix well; stir the strawberries into the mixture.
Strawberry Orange Sauce: Blend or process strawberries and juice until smooth; strain.
Serves 4.

Approximately 505 kilojoules (121 calories) per serve.

COTTAGE APPLE PUDDING

This recipe is unsuitable to freeze or microwave.

1 medium apple (150g), finely chopped
1 teaspoon lemon juice
2 teaspoons Sweetaddin
¼ teaspoon ground cinnamon
½ cup skim milk
¼ cup low-fat cottage cheese (60g)
1 egg, lightly beaten
2 teaspoons Sweetaddin, extra
4 slices wholemeal bread

Combine apple in a bowl with lemon juice, Sweetaddin and cinnamon. Combine milk and cheese in another bowl, stir in egg and extra Sweetaddin. Cut from each slice of bread a circle large enough to cover base of each of 4 ovenproof dishes (three-quarter cup capacity). Top bread with half the cottage cheese mixture, top with apple mixture, then remaining cottage cheese mixture. Bake in a moderate oven for about 30 minutes. Serve hot or cold and sprinkle with a little extra cinnamon, if preferred.
Serves 4.

Approximately 525 kilojoules (125 calories) per serve.

BOYSENBERRY APPLE CRUMBLE

Fresh or frozen berries can be used in this dish. This recipe is not suitable to freeze or microwave.

200g boysenberries
1 large apple (200g), chopped
3 teaspoons sugar
CRUMBLE TOPPING
⅓ cup untoasted muesli (40g)
1 tablespoon plain flour
2 teaspoons brown sugar
30g butter

Combine berries, apple and sugar in saucepan, bring to the boil, reduce heat, simmer, uncovered, until apple is just tender.

Divide berry mixture evenly into 4 ovenproof dishes (three-quarter cup capacity), sprinkle with topping. Bake in moderate oven for about 15 minutes or until browned.
Crumble Topping: Combine muesli, flour and sugar in bowl, rub in butter.
Serves 4.

Approximately 655 kilojoules (156 calories) per serve.

ABOVE: Strawberry and Orange Crepes.
RIGHT: Top: Boysenberry Apple Crumble; bottom: Cottage Apple Pudding

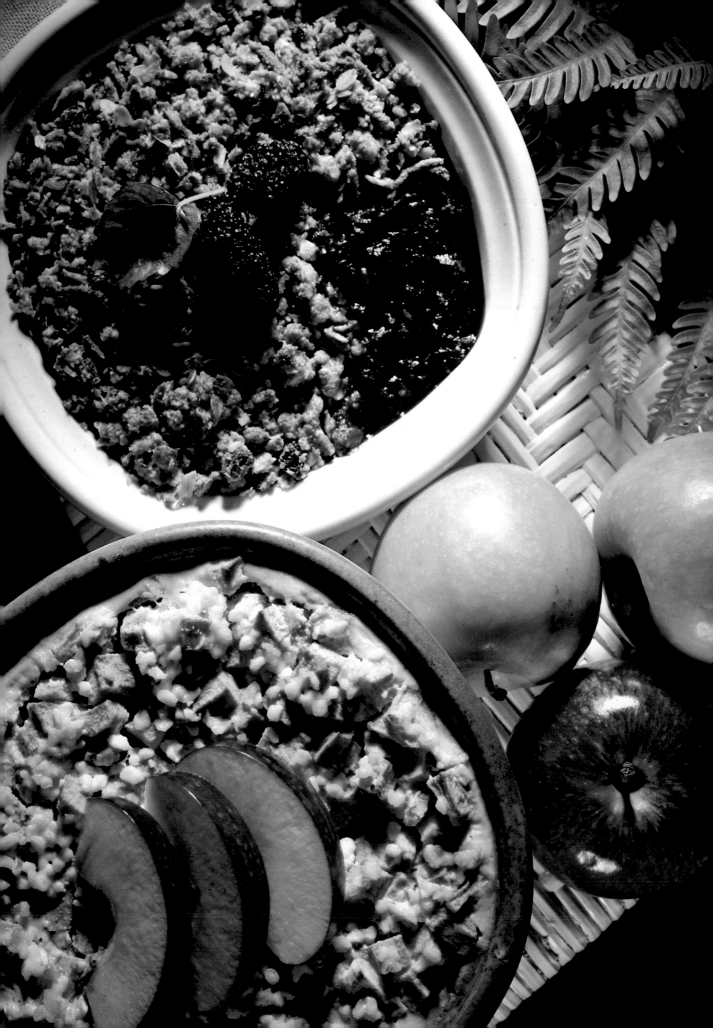

PEACHY STRAWBERRY AND APPLE JELLIES

Jellies can be made up to a day ahead; keep, covered, in refrigerator. This recipe is not suitable to freeze.

3 teaspoons gelatine
2 tablespoons water
¾ cup unsweetened clear apple juice
250g punnet strawberries, sliced
4 fresh peaches (480g), chopped

Sprinkle gelatine over water, dissolve over hot water (or microwave on HIGH for about 20 seconds), cool to room temperature. Combine gelatine and apple juice in bowl, pour 1 tablespoon of the apple mixture into 4 serving dishes (half cup capacity), refrigerate until set.

Arrange some of the strawberries over apple mixture; top with peaches, then remaining strawberries. Pour remaining apple mixture into dishes. Refrigerate several hours or until set.

Serves 4.

Approximately 340 kilojoules (81 calories) per serve.

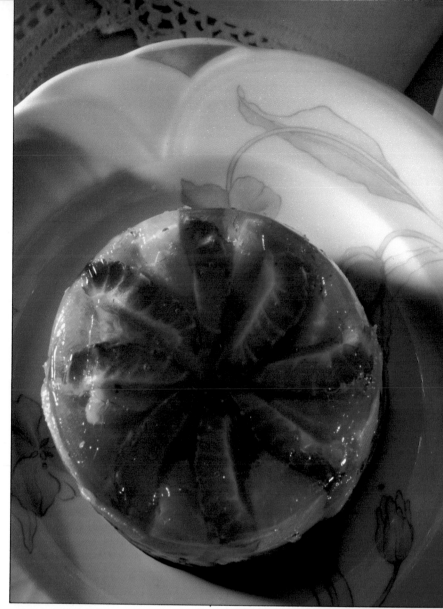

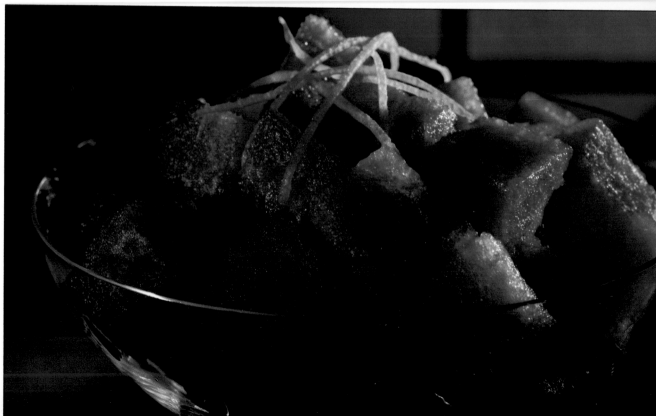

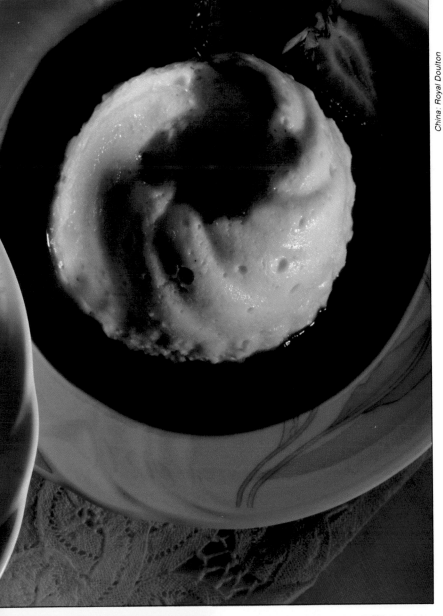

China: Royal Doulton

LEMON CHEESE DESSERTS WITH STRAWBERRY SAUCE

Desserts can be made up to 2 days ahead; keep, covered, in refrigerator. This recipe is not suitable to freeze.

¾ cup ricotta cheese (150g)
⅓ cup sour light cream
2 tablespoons Sweetaddin
2 teaspoons grated lemon rind
1 teaspoon gelatine
1 tablespoon lemon juice
2 egg whites
STRAWBERRY SAUCE
250g punnet strawberries
2 teaspoons lemon juice
1 tablespoon Sweetaddin

Sieve cheese into bowl, stir in cream, Sweetaddin and rind. Sprinkle gelatine over lemon juice, dissolve over hot water (or microwave on HIGH for about 20 seconds), cool 5 minutes before stirring into cheese mixture.

Beat egg whites until soft peaks form, fold into cheese mixture. Spoon mixture into 4 greased dishes (one-third cup capacity), refrigerate several hours or until set. Turn onto serving plates, top with sauce.

Strawberry Sauce: Blend or process all ingredients until smooth.

Serves 4.

Approximately 595 kilojoules (142 calories) per serve.

VANILLA ICE-CREAM

This is a good basic ice-cream which makes enough for about 12 half cup serves. We served our ice-cream with puréed raspberries; use fruit of your choice, but remember to count the extra kilojoules. Ice-cream can be made a week ahead; keep, covered, in freezer.

¼ cup castor sugar (60g)
¼ cup water
1 teaspoon gelatine
⅔ cup skim milk powder (80g)
2 cups skim milk
1 teaspoon white vinegar
1 teaspoon vanilla essence

Combine sugar and water in a small saucepan, add gelatine, stir constantly over heat without boiling until sugar and gelatine are dissolved. Transfer mixture to small bowl, whisk in powdered milk, then gradually beat in skim milk with electric mixer. Pour into 2 lamington pans; cover with foil, freeze for about 1 hour or until almost set.

Transfer mixture to medium bowl, add vinegar and essence, beat with electric mixer until thick and creamy. Return to lamington pans, cover, freeze for about 3 hours or overnight.

Makes about 1½ litres (6 cups).

Approximately 250 kilojoules (60 calories) per serve.

Glass dish: Sasaki from Dansab; plate: Villeroy & Boch

CHILLED HONEY WATERMELON

Recipe unsuitable to freeze.

⅓ cup lemon juice
1 tablespoon honey
4 cups watermelon chunks (1kg)

Combine lemon juice and honey in a bowl, add watermelon, mix gently. Cover, refrigerate for at least 1 hour before serving.

Serves 4.

Approximately 325 kilojoules (77 calories) per serve.

LEFT: Chilled Honey Watermelon.
ABOVE: Left: Peachy Strawberry and Apple Jellies; right: Lemon Cheese Desserts with Strawberry Sauce

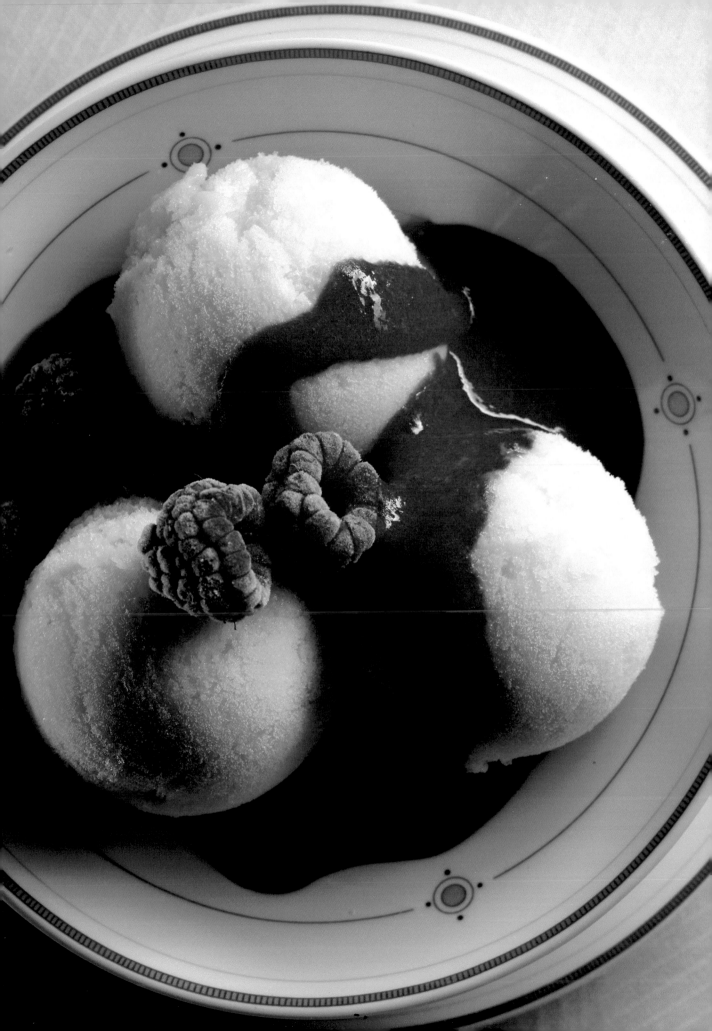

MANGO GINGER SORBET

Sorbet can be made up to 3 days ahead; keep, covered, in freezer. This recipe makes about 4 three-quarter cup serves.

1½ cups water
¼ cup sugar (60g)
2 small mangoes (400g)
2 tablespoons lemon juice
2 teaspoons chopped glacé ginger
2 egg whites

Combine water and sugar in saucepan, stir constantly over heat, without boiling, until sugar is dissolved. Bring to the boil, boil 10 minutes, uncovered, without stirring, cool, refrigerate until syrup is cold.

Blend or process mango flesh, lemon juice and ginger until smooth, add sugar syrup, process until well combined. Pour mixture into lamington pan, cover with foil, freeze for about 1 hour or until partly set.

Process mango mixture with egg whites until smooth, return mixture to lamington pan, cover, freeze several hours or until set.

Makes about 3 cups.

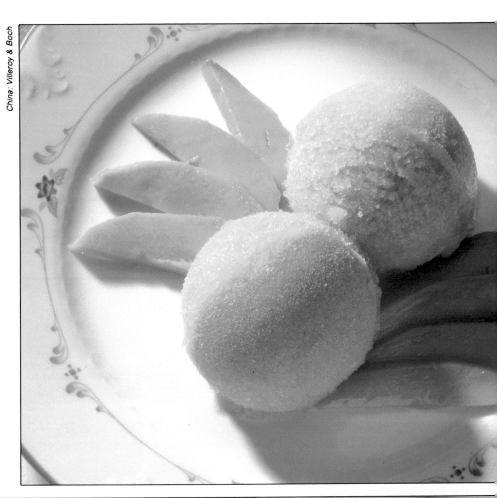

Approximately 555 kilojoules (132 calories) per serve.

LEFT: Vanilla Ice-Cream. RIGHT: Mango Ginger Sorbet. BELOW: Left: Creamy Strawberry Treats; right: Rainbow Delights

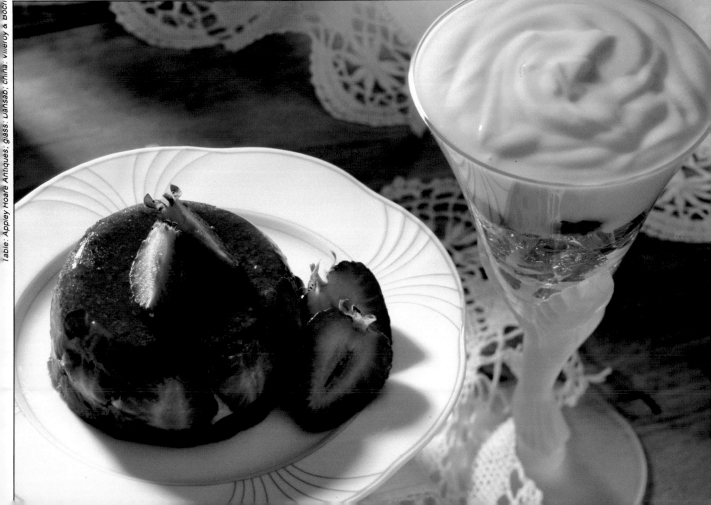

CREAMY STRAWBERRY TREATS

Treats can be made a day ahead. This recipe is not suitable to freeze.

250g punnet strawberries
2 teaspoons castor sugar
200g carton low-fat plain yoghurt
1 tablespoon castor sugar, extra
2 tablespoons cream
3 teaspoons gelatine
1 tablespoon water

Slice 4 strawberries thinly, arrange around sides of 4 individual dishes (half cup capacity). Blend or process remaining strawberries and sugar until smooth; transfer to bowl.

Combine yoghurt in another bowl with extra sugar and cream.

Sprinkle gelatine over water, dissolve over hot water (or microwave on HIGH for about 20 seconds), cool, do not allow to set.

Add half the gelatine mixture to the strawberry mixture and the remaining half to the yoghurt mixture. Divide half the strawberry mixture between the prepared dishes, refrigerate until almost set. Pour yoghurt mixture evenly over strawberry layer, refrigerate until almost set. Top with remaining strawberry mixture, refrigerate until set.

Serves 4.

Approximately 490 kilojoules (117 calories) per serve.

RAINBOW DELIGHTS

Jelly and custard can be prepared the day before required. Store, covered, in refrigerator. This recipe is not suitable to freeze.

9g sachet low-joule passionfruit and
**   mango jelly**
425g can sweet red cherries,
**   drained, stoned**
VANILLA CUSTARD
375ml can evaporated skim milk
1 egg, lightly beaten
¼ cup castor sugar (60g)
1 tablespoon plain flour
¼ cup water
2 teaspoons vanilla essence

Make jelly as instructed on packet, pour into lamington pan, cool, refrigerate until set.

Chop jelly roughly, spoon into serving dishes, top with cherries then custard; refrigerate before serving.

Vanilla Custard: Combine milk, egg, sugar and blended flour and water in a saucepan, stir constantly over heat until mixture boils and thickens. Stir in essence, cover surface of custard with plastic wrap to prevent skin forming, cool to room temperature.

Serves 4.

Approximately 920 kilojoules (220 calories) per serve.

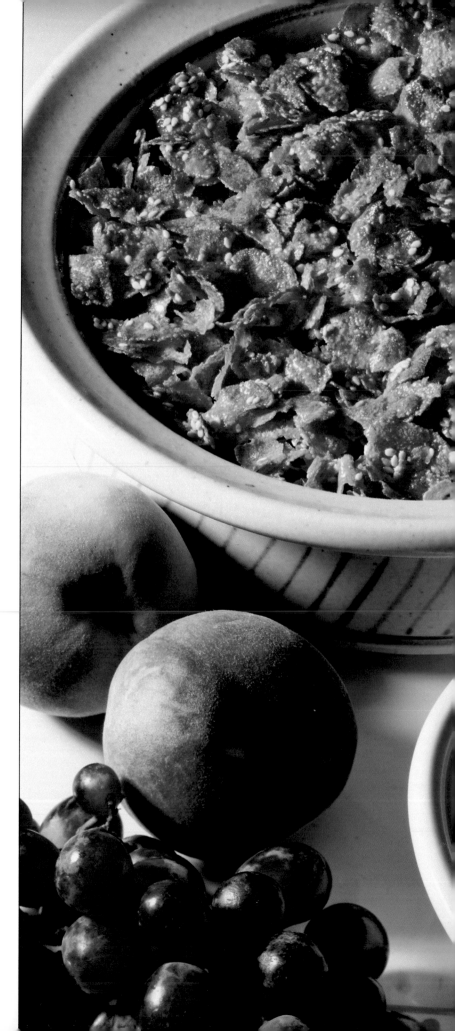

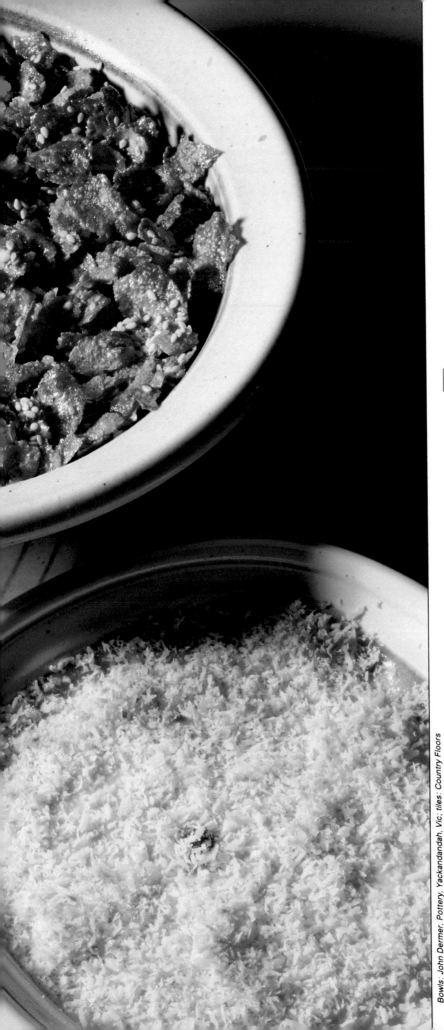

PEACH SULTANA CRUNCH

Recipe unsuitable to freeze.

**425g can unsweetened sliced
   peaches**
½ cup sultanas (80g)
½ teaspoon ground cinnamon
15g butter
1 tablespoon honey
1½ cups cornflakes (45g)
3 teaspoons sesame seeds

Drain peaches, reserve half cup syrup.

Combine peaches, syrup, sultanas and cinnamon in a bowl, spread into ovenproof dish (4 cup capacity).

Melt butter and honey in a saucepan (or microwave on HIGH for about 1 minute), stir in cornflakes and sesame seeds. Spread mixture evenly over the peaches and bake in moderate oven for about 20 minutes or until golden brown (or microwave on HIGH for about 4 minutes).

Serves 4.

Approximately 785 kilojoules (187 calories) per serve.

COCONUT BREAD PUDDING

This recipe is unsuitable to freeze or microwave.

2 eggs
1 tablespoon castor sugar
½ teaspoon coconut essence
⅓ cup canned reduced cream
⅔ cup skim milk
1 slice white bread
1 tablespoon sultanas
1 tablespoon coconut

Combine eggs, sugar and essence in bowl, whisk until combined; gradually whisk in cream and milk.

Remove and discard crusts from bread, cut bread into small cubes. Place bread cubes into an ovenproof dish (3 cup capacity), sprinkle evenly with sultanas, top with custard mixture. Place dish into baking dish with enough hot water to come half way up the sides of dish. Bake in moderate oven for 30 minutes.

Sprinkle custard evenly with coconut, return to oven further 10 minutes, or until pudding is set. Stand 5 minutes before serving. Serve warm or cold.

Serves 4.

Approximately 675 kilojoules (161 calories) per serve.

Bowls: John Dermer, Pottery, Yackandandah, Vic; tiles: Country Floors

Top: Peach Sultana Crunch; bottom: Coconut Bread Pudding

121

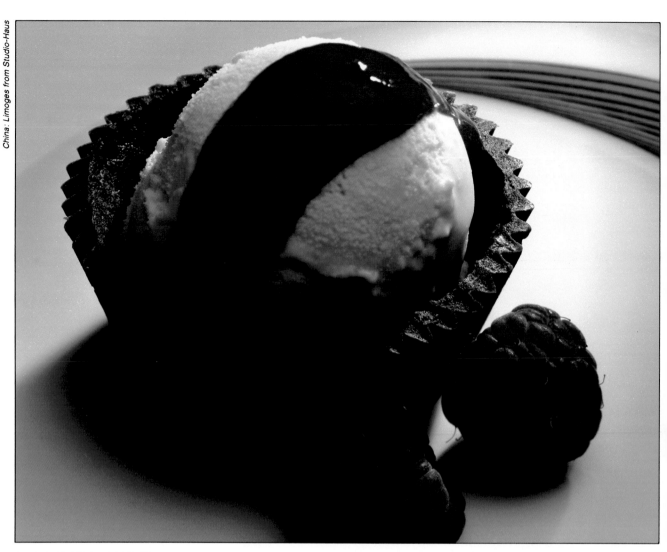

CHOCOLATE BASKETS

You will need to make 4 chocolate cases for this recipe. First make moulds by placing 3 paper patty cases inside each other to give the strength required to hold the chocolate. Chocolate cases can be made up to a week ahead; store in an airtight container in the refrigerator. This recipe is not suitable to freeze.

2 tablespoons icing sugar
3 teaspoons cocoa
30g Copha, melted
½ teaspoon vanilla essence
low kilojoule ice-cream
RASPBERRY SAUCE
¾ cup raspberries (90g)
2 teaspoons Sweetaddin
2 teaspoons lemon juice

Combine sifted icing sugar and cocoa in a bowl, stir in Copha and essence. Spread chocolate mixture over side and base of each set of paper patty cases, refrigerate until serving time.

Peel paper patty cases carefully from chocolate, place cases on serving plates. Place a small scoop of ice-cream (about a quarter of a cup) into each case, top with raspberry sauce.
Raspberry Sauce: Blend or process all ingredients until smooth.

Serves 4.

Approximately 730 kilojoules (174 calories) per serve.

BANANA COCONUT FREEZE

Recipe can be made up to 3 days ahead, keep, covered, in freezer. This recipe makes about 8 half cup serves.

340ml can coconut milk
1 cup skim milk
2 eggs
¼ cup castor sugar (60g)
2 teaspoons gelatine
¼ cup water
1 medium ripe banana (150g),
    mashed

Whisk coconut milk, skim milk, eggs and sugar together in heatproof bowl or double saucepan over simmering water until warm and frothy.

Sprinkle gelatine over water, dissolve over hot water (or microwave on HIGH about 20 seconds), cool, do not allow to set. Gradually whisk gelatine mixture into egg mixture, pour into lamington pan, cover with foil, freeze several hours or until set.

Chop mixture roughly, place in large bowl, beat with electric mixer until light and fluffy; beat in banana. Return mixture to lamington pan, cover, freeze several hours or until set.

Makes about 1 litre (4 cups).

Approximately 740 kilojoules (177 calories) per serve.

ABOVE: Chocolate Baskets.
RIGHT: Banana Coconut Freeze

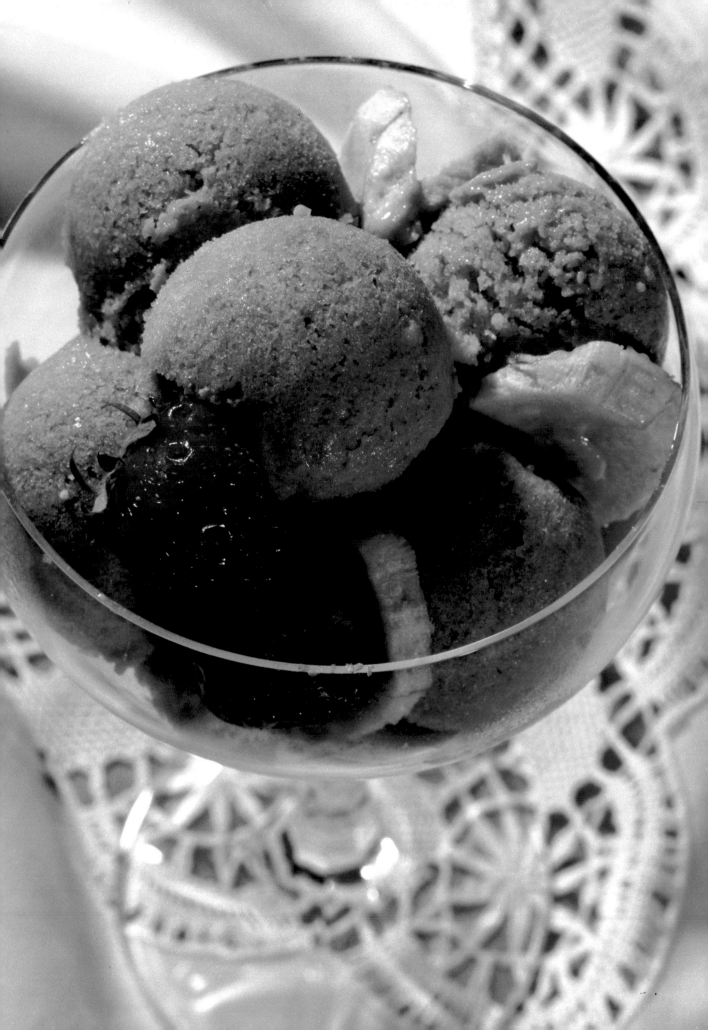

GLOSSARY

This helpful information explains some of the terms used in this book, including differences that can occur in the names of ingredients.

BACON
Rashers: bacon slices.

BEANS
Black beans: fermented, salted soya beans. Use either canned or dried; one can be substituted for the other. Drain and rinse the canned variety, soak and rinse the dried variety. Leftover beans will keep well for months in an airtight jar in the refrigerator. Mash beans when cooking to release the flavour.

GREEN BEANS: French beans.

BEEF
Eye fillet: tenderloin.
Mince: ground beef.

BEETROOT: ordinary round beet.

BICARBONATE OF SODA: baking soda, a component of baking powder.

BISCUIT CRUMBS, SWEET: use any plain, sweet biscuits (cookies). Blend or process biscuits until finely and evenly crushed.

BLANCHING: usually required when the cooking of the food is minimal, as in snow peas or spinach, or when an ingredient needs to be cooked lightly before a longer cooking process takes place. This is often the case before vegetables are stir-fried.
To blanch a vegetable: bring a pan of water to the boil, add the specified ingredient, then follow individual recipe instructions.

BOUILLON: see Stock.

BREADCRUMBS
Stale: use 1 or 2 day old white or wholemeal bread made into crumbs by grating, blending or processing.
Dry: use packaged breadcrumbs.

BUTTER: use salted or unsalted (sweet) butter depending on your diet, or use margarine of your choice. The kilojoule count is the same for both margarine and butter. 125g butter is equal to 1 stick butter.

BUTTERNUT PUMPKIN: any type of pumpkin can be substituted.

CHEESE
Cottage cheese: we used low-fat cottage cheese with less than 4 percent fat content.
Fetta cheese: we used cheese with 15 percent fat content.
Mozzarella cheese: we used cheese with 25 percent fat content.
Parmesan cheese: we used cheese with 30 percent fat content.
Ricotta cheese: we used cheese with 10 percent fat content.
Tasty cheese: use a firm, good-tasting cheddar cheese. We used cheese with 33 percent fat content.

CHICKEN
Breast fillets: skinless and boneless.
Breast on the bone: sold either whole or as half breasts, usually with skin.
Drumsticks: leg with skin intact.
Marylands: joined leg and thigh with skin intact.
Thigh fillets: skinless and boneless.

CHILLIES, FRESH: are available in many different types and sizes. The small ones (bird's eye or bird peppers) are the hottest. Use tight-fitting gloves when handling and chopping fresh chillies as they can burn your skin. The seeds are the hottest part of the chillies, so remove them if you want to reduce the heat content of recipes.

COD, SMOKED: smoked whitefish.

COPHA: a solid white shortening based on coconut oil. No known substitute outside Australia.

CORNFLOUR: cornstarch.

CREAM
Pouring cream: light cream or half 'n' half with 33 to 35 percent fat content.
Reduced cream: a canned product with 25 percent fat content.
Sour light cream: a light, commercially cultured sour cream with 18 percent fat content.

EGGPLANT: aubergine.

ENGLISH SPINACH: see Spinach.

ESSENCE: extract.

FLOUR
Plain flour: all-purpose flour.
Self-raising flour: substitute plain (all-purpose) flour and baking powder in the proportion of three-quarters metric cup plain flour to 2 level metric teaspoons baking powder, sift together several times before using. If using an 8oz measuring cup, use 1 cup plain flour to 2 level metric teaspoons baking powder.

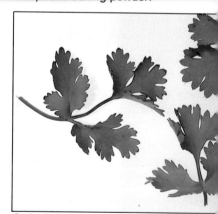
Coriander

OVEN TEMPERATURES

Electric Temperatures	Celsius	Fahrenheit	Gas Temperatures	Celsius	Fahrenheit
Very slow	120	250	Very slow	120	250
Slow	150	300	Slow	150	300
Moderately slow	160-180	325-350	Moderately slow	160	325
Moderate	180-200	375-400	Moderate	180	350
Moderately hot	210-230	425-450	Moderately hot	190	375
Hot	240-250	475-500	Hot	200	400
Very hot	260	525-550	Very hot	230	450

FRENCH DRESSING: we used Kraft Light No Oil French Dressing in our recipes. Recipe given below is a good substitute; three-quarters of a cup is about 9 tablespoons, there are about 25 kilojoules (6 calories) in each tablespoon of dressing.

Slimmer's French Dressing
¼ cup white vinegar
¼ cup lemon juice
¼ cup water
1 small chicken stock cube, crumbled
1 clove garlic, crushed
1 tablespoon chopped fresh chives
½ teaspoon dry mustard
2 teaspoons sugar
Combine all ingredients in a screw-top jar, shake well. Makes ¾ cup.

GHERKIN: cornichon.

GINGER
Fresh ginger: ginger root.
Glacé ginger: crystallised ginger can be substituted; rinse off the sugar with warm water, dry ginger well before using.

GREASING: use a commercial non-stick spray to grease pans when possible or to eliminate or decrease oil or butter in recipes.

GRILL, GRILLER: broil, broiler.

HERBS: we have specified when to use fresh or dried herbs. We used dried (not ground) herbs in the proportion of 1:4 for fresh herbs; for example, 1 teaspoon dried herbs instead of 4 teaspoons (1 tablespoon) chopped fresh herbs.

Basil

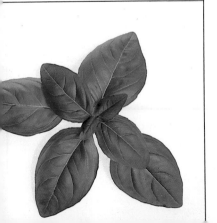

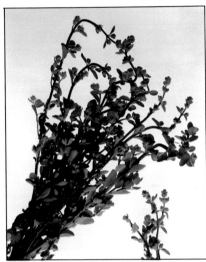

Oregano

JALAPENO CHILLIES: imported, canned, pickled, hot chillies. Store any leftover chillies in their liquid in an airtight container in the refrigerator.

KIWI FRUIT: Chinese gooseberry.

KUMARA: a variety of sweet potato, orange in colour.

LAMB
Chump chops: chops cut from the chump section, between the leg and the mid-loin.
Cutlets: chops cut from the rib loin.
Loin chops: chops cut from the mid-loin below the rib loin.
Racks: joined cutlets from rib loin.
Shanks: cut from the forelegs.

LAMINGTON PAN: a rectangular slab pan with a depth of about 4cm.

LETTUCE: we used mostly iceberg, radicchio, mignonette and butter lettuce; any variety can be used.

MAYONNAISE: we used a low-oil commercial mayonnaise with 12 percent fat content.

MILK
Evaporated skim milk: canned milk with 0.3 percent fat content.
Skim milk: we used milk with 0.1 percent fat content.
Skim milk powder: we used dried milk powder with 1 percent fat content when dry and 0.1 percent when reconstituted.

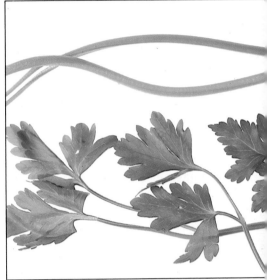

Continental Parsley

MUESLI: granola.

MUSSEL MEAT: available from most fishmongers. If unavailable, buy double the weight required in recipe of mussels in their shells. Cook in boiling water (or microwave on HIGH) for a minute or two or until they open. Discard any unopened shells.

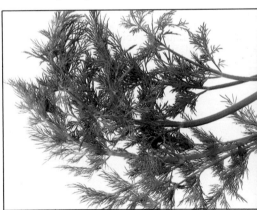

Dill

MUSTARD, SEEDED: a French style of textured mustard with crushed mustard seeds.

NUTS: packaged ground almonds or hazelnuts; we used commercially ground nuts, unless otherwise specified in recipes.

OIL: light polyunsaturated salad oil.

OYSTER SAUCE: a rich, brown bottled sauce made from oysters, cooked in salt and soya sauce.

PEAS, SNOW: also known as mange tout, sugar peas or Chinese peas, they are small flat pods with barely formed peas; they are eaten whole. You need only to top and tail young pods, older ones need stringing. Cook for a short time (about 30 seconds) either by stir-frying or blanching, or until tender-crisp.

PEPPERS: Capsicum or bell peppers.

PIMENTO: allspice.

PIMIENTOS: canned or bottled whole or halved peppers.

PORK
Butterfly: skinless, boneless mid-loin chop which has been split in half and opened out flat.
Fillets: skinless, boneless eye-fillet from the loin.
Steaks: schnitzels, usually cut from the leg or rump.

PUNNET: basket usually holding about 250g fruit.

ROCKMELON: cantaloupe.

SCALLOPS: we used the scallops with coral (roe) attached. Saucer scallops, found in northern Australian waters, are commonly used in restaurants and are sometimes available in fish markets. They can be substituted in any of these recipes.

SHALLOTS
Golden shallots: a member of the onion family, with a delicate onion/garlic flavour.
Green shallots: known as spring onions in some Australian States, scallions in some other countries.

SOYA SAUCE: made from fermented soya beans; we used 2 types, the light and dark variety. The light sauce is generally used with white meat

Left: Green shallots; right: golden shallots

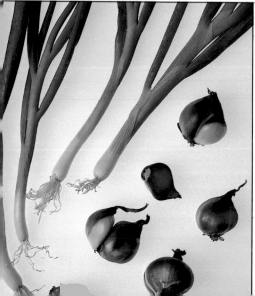

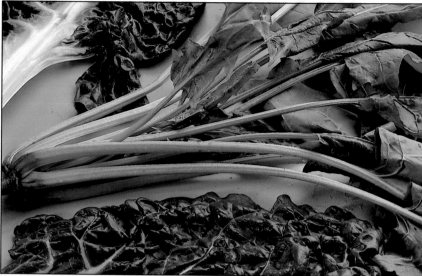

Top: Silver beet; centre: English spinach

dishes, and the darker variety with red meat dishes, but this is only a guide. Dark soya is generally used for colour, and the light for flavour. Light soya sauce has more salt than dark.

SPINACH
English spinach: a soft-leafed vegetable, more delicate in taste than silver beet (spinach); tender silver beet can be substituted for English spinach in most recipes.
Silver beet: a large-leafed vegetable, remove white stalk and discard.

STOCK: a small stock cube is equivalent to 1 teaspoon powdered bouillon (stock powder).

>**To make your own stock:** use chicken, veal or beef bones with vegetables such as carrots, celery and onions. Place all these in a saucepan with enough water to cover the ingredients. Cover the pan, bring to the boil, reduce heat, simmer, covered, for about 1 hour for chicken; 2 hours for veal and beef. Cool to room temperature, strain; refrigerate the stock overnight. Next day, remove the fat with an egg slide and discard.

To freeze the stock: boil the stock until it is reduced by about half. Cool, freeze in measured amounts — usually 1 cup (250ml) for easy future use. Remember to add more water when using the stock in recipes, to reconstitute the liquid. 250ml of home-made stock would contain about 100 kilojoules (25 calories).

SUGAR: we used a coarse granulated table sugar unless otherwise stated.
Castor: fine granulated table sugar.
Brown: soft, brown sugar.
Icing: confectioners, or powdered, sugar. We used the icing sugar mixture, not pure icing sugar.
Raw: natural, light granulated sugar.

SULTANAS: seedless white raisins.

SWEETENERS
Liquid: we used 2 brands, Sugarine and Hermesetas. Both are about the same in strength; 4 drops are equal to 1 teaspoon sugar in taste. 1 teaspoon of the liquid is equal to about half cup sugar in taste. You can use any liquid sweetener; read the label and adjust the amounts to make the strength equal to the amounts we used.
Powdered: we used 2 brands, Sweetaddin and Sugarsweet. 1 teaspoon of each of these ingredients contains about 4 kilojoules (1 calorie). Check kilojoules on package. These sweeteners are available in pharmacies and most supermarkets.

TERIYAKI SAUCE: a sauce based on the lighter Japanese soya sauce; it contains sugar, spices and vinegar.

TOMATO PUREE: known as tomato sauce in some other countries. You can use canned tomato purée or a purée of fresh, ripe tomatoes made by blending or processing the required amount for the recipe.

TOMATO SAUCE: tomato ketchup.

VEAL
Cutlets: cut from the rib and loin.
Steaks: schnitzels, cut from the leg.
Chops: cut from the rib and loin.

VEGERONI: vegetable-flavoured, multi-coloured pasta.

WATER CRACKERS: plain crackers.

WHITE FISH: simply means non-oily fish, and could include bream, flathead, whiting, snapper, jewfish and ling. Redfish comes into this category.

WHOLEMEAL: wholewheat.

YOGHURT: we used low-fat plain yoghurt with about 0.2 percent fat.

ZUCCHINI: courgette.

INDEX

Production editor: Maryanne Blacker
Art director: Robbylee Phelan
Deputy editor: Enid Morrison
Sub-editor: Mary-Anne Danah
Editorial assistant: Louise McGeachie

Photographers: Paul Clarke
Ashley Mackeviciu
Andre Martin
Luis Martin

Publisher: Richard Walsh
Associate publisher: Sally Milner
Editor-in-chief: Dawn Swain

Food editor: Pamela Clark
Assistant food editor: Barbara Northwoo
Chief home economist: Jan Castorina
Home economists: John Allen
Wendy Berecry
Jane Ash
Karen Green
Sue Hipwell
Louise Sakiris
Kathy Wharton

Food stylists: Jacqui Hing
Carolyn Fienberg
Rosemary Ingram
Editorial assistant: Denise Prentice
Kitchen assistant: Amy Wong